Astrology & Weight Control
The Jupiter/Pluto Connection

by Beverly Flynn

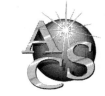

ACS Publications
San Diego, California

International Standard Book Number 0-935127-91-7

Printed in the United States of America.

Published by ACS Publications
5521 Ruffin Road
San Diego, California 92123

First Printing, July 2003

To Cicely,
my friend for all seasons.

Table of Contents

INTRODUCTION

Once upon a time, in a faraway land, there lived a beautiful princess (or handsome prince, whatever the case may be), who was burdened with seventy-five extra pounds of the most obstinate, tenacious, malicious fat ever. This fat was a "gift" from an evil spell cast upon the princess some several thousand years earlier by a vindictive and venomous sorcerer who, in retaliation for the princess' rebuff of his attentions, sentenced her to an eternity of enormity unless she could discover the true secret of fat.

"Eat, eat, eat, and never know why,
Until your presence covers the sky.
Unlock the mystery of the cursed weight,
Thence lay it down and change your fate."

And thus the spell was cast.

So, for thousands of years, the princess dragged her uncomfortable, overweight body from town to town, kingdom to kingdom, searching for anyone who could assist her in solving the mystery of fat. She met many people on this journey, people who claimed to be able to help her, but who, in fact, only made her situation worse.

"You need a magic potion," they would tell her. "Bat wings and frog eyes," they usually recommended, "and a huge dose of blood from this or that." She tried them all, the bitter potions, the smelly potions, the ones that tickled her nose as she drank them, and the ones that made her hair stand on end, but to no avail. None of them worked and so she kept searching.

In her travels, she met the timeless old woman from the village of Dietville, who promised her that she could rid herself of her unwanted weight if she followed a special secret eating plan.

"I beseech you," the old woman told her in a very shrill voice, "follow the eating rules I give you and you will rid yourself of all your unwanted weight." The old woman handed the princess a stone upon which were etched the names of the only foods she could eat and the portion sizes. "You cannot deviate from the plan," the old woman warned sternly, "for if you eat just one bite of any forbidden food, you will not lose a single pound."

So the princess faithfully followed the secret, special eating plan, and it did allow her to shed fifty pounds. But as soon as she began to eat normal food, she regained those same pounds plus an additional sixty. Special diets were not the answer, she discovered. So she kept searching.

During her travels, she met a magician from the town of Willpower, who told her that all it takes is inner strength and resolution to lose those extra pounds, and that she simply needed to develop the right frame of mind.

"I will teach you how to develop a mind so strong and a will so purposeful, that you can overcome any obstacle and defeat any foe."

So the princess took lessons from the magician on developing strength of mind, and she applied this knowledge to her weight problem. However, she discovered that her will was not strong enough to rid herself of the unwanted poundage, and so not only was she doomed to carry the extra weight, but now she added to it guilt and a sense of failure.

This went on for many, many centuries, the lovely princess traveling from town to town, trying new diets, drinking stranger and stranger potions, only to become larger and larger. Then one day, the depressed and ever-expanding princess was walking beside a river and encountered a pointy-eared elf named Sebastian. Sebastian told her that she would never successfully lose her extra weight through diet, exercise, or willpower alone, and that potions, no matter what they contained, would not work. He told her that he knew the answer to the mystery of fat that she had been searching for all these years, and that he could teach her, but only on one condition.

"And what might the condition be?" the tired princess asked skeptically, suspecting that he wanted gold or some other material reward.

"All I ask," replied Sebastian, "is that once you learn the secret, you pass it on to someone else who is also searching for the truth."

This seemed like a fair request. So the princess sat down on a large rock beside the river and listened to the little elf.

And this is what he told her.

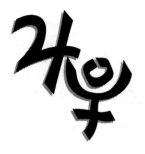

CHAPTER ONE

UNDERSTANDING JUPITER, THE ENLIGHTENER

Significance: 1 a: something that is conveyed as a meaning often obscurely or indirectly **b:** the quality of conveying or implying **2 a:** the quality of being important: MOMENT **b:** the quality of being statistically significant

This book is about significances. That word will appear many times in this writing because it is the essence of what I am trying to convey. It's very difficult for most twenty-first century beings to understand the importance of looking for the deeper meaning in any given situation. We are all accustomed to thinking narrowly and superficially. We believe only what we can verify with our senses in the physical world. If we can't see, touch, hear, taste or smell it, it isn't real to us and therefore has no meaning. This book is going to try to change that mindset.

The idea that everything we see manifested in the physical world has a deeper meaning is not a new one. In fact, basic astrology is based on that tenet. We learn in astrology that all the planets and signs have specific meanings, and that those meanings manifest in our lives in a variety of ways. Carrying that idea a step further, each of the planets has a symbolic significance, which manifests both outwardly and inwardly. That is, each planet correlates with certain obvious physical expressions and also with less obvious parts of our lives.

So, as an example, let's look at a person with Mars squaring Uranus in the natal chart. Ostensibly, this combination of energies of Mars and Uranus often manifests, or appears, in the physical world as someone with an explosive temper, and/or someone who is accident-prone. But the hidden or esoteric meaning of this aspect is that of incorrect use or incorrect placement of the energies symbolized by these planets. Mars represents our tremendous vitality to accomplish goals, but if we don't direct this vitality towards the appropriate goal, then all this wonderful energy becomes a detriment instead of an attribute. The person with Mars square Uranus has to learn his true soul path and use his immense storehouse of Martian energies to that end. Once he has done that, through his own efforts he will be able to transform his violent temper and tendency towards accidents into energetic, directed purpose.

Let's look at another example. One of the visible manifestations of Saturn trining Venus in the natal chart is someone with a very stable marriage. Saturn, after all, is the planet that indicates form and stability, and Venus symbolizes love and partnerships. But the underlying, or hidden meaning of this trine is that this person intuitively understands the idea of right relationships, as these concepts are deeply ingrained in this person's psyche. The Venus trine Saturn individual has mastered the lessons of love and relationships, and has therefore earned the right to a stable and loving marriage because they are responsible, committed and loving in their approach to all relationships.

This concept of a dual meaning for all manifested effects can be stated in many ways. Throughout this book, you will see me using various pairs and combinations of words, such as obvious and hidden, ostensible and esoteric, objective and subjective, apparent and intrinsic, visible and invisible, to describe this idea of an effect and its underlying meaning or significance. You can probably come up with many more pairs of words and phrases to express this relationship between the seen and the unseen, but these examples are enough to convey the meaning for now. The main thing is that you understand the concept, because it is basic in understanding the role of astrology in weight control.

It has been my experience that the planets Jupiter and Pluto both have major significance in regard to personal weight, objectively and subjectively. There are definite, specific effects that can be seen, and definite, obscure and intangible effects that need to be analyzed for their esoteric or hidden meaning. Excess weight represents something more than just excess weight. It has an underlying meaning, or significance. That is why, by doing an in-depth study of Jupiter and Pluto, we can arrive at some conclusions regarding the visible and invisible effects of the motifs represented by these two planets, and can then use that information to work both objectively and subjectively on our own weight issues.

Before we begin our study of Jupiter and Pluto, though, let's review some astrological basics.

WHAT IS ASTROLOGY?

The universe is a marvelous and, at the same time, mind boggling place. In order to guide us through the maze that is life, the universe has provided us with several tools. The science of astrology is one of these tools, and through its study, we can learn the answers to many of our questions, and therefore find that needed sense of direction so that we no longer feel lost. Through the study of astrology, we learn how to interpret the meanings of the planets and their geometric relationships and to extrapolate that information which will help us in our own lives. Astrology is the universal compass that aids humanity in its journey towards self-knowledge and soul growth.

As above so below, we are told, which implies that humanity can learn to imitate the activities of the larger universe, albeit it on a smaller scale. The greater and more important implication is that even though we have a very long way to go, we too can reach our greatest potential, and that we can eventually tap into the divinity in ourselves, no matter how deeply it is buried. Astrology is a tool that has been given to us to assist us in our journey towards this self-realization, towards that quest for our inner divinity.

Even though humanity has been practicing the science of astrology for thousands of years, it is a science that is still in its infancy. It is constantly growing and changing as new planets and asteroids are being discovered. But it is helpful to us at every stage of its development. As we learn more about the universe, we also learn more about astrology and, in turn, we learn more about ourselves.

We already discussed the fact that each of the planets in our solar system represents different issues and needs and these drives affect various areas of our lives. But why is it important that we study them? Well, for one thing, learning to identify these motives and the way they affect us will allow us to identify and catalog our strengths and weaknesses. Knowing which tools we came into the world with enables us to know how best to approach life and how to fulfill our destinies. By studying the planets and their significance in our individual charts, we are able to tap into the appropriate energies at the appropriate times. It is a very useful science, a gift from the universe, and it would be foolish to ignore it.

Astrology mainly concerns itself with ten planets, twelve astrological signs and twelve houses. Considering the Earth as the center of our little universe, since that's where we are located, the "planets" in our solar system are the Sun, the Moon, Mercury, Venus, Mars, Jupiter, Saturn, Uranus, Neptune and Pluto. Jupiter and Pluto, as I pointed out earlier, are the planets that have the most to do with weight, as Jupiter is the planet of expansion, and Pluto is the planet of elimination. But what does that mean?

To answer that question, we are going to really get to know these two planets. I'm going to present a lot of information regarding Jupiter in this chapter, and in the next chapter, I will do the same for Pluto. Some of the information may seem irrelevant, or extraneous. But please bear with me. Later on in the book we will pull it all together, and you will see the relevance.

JUPITER: THE EPITOME OF LARGE

Jupiter is enormous. Jupiter is the largest planet in our solar system, so it would make sense that it should have something to do with largeness and weight. Its diameter at its equator is about 88,700 miles. Indeed, the diameter of the planet is eleven times that of our Earth. In addition, it would take about 1,300 Earths to fill up the volume of this gigantic planet.

Jupiter has a greater mass than any of the other planets in our solar system. The definition of mass in Webster's Dictionary is a quantity or aggregate of matter usually of considerable size, which is quite appropriate for our subject matter. However, another, even more appropriate definition, again according to Webster's, is as follows:

"The property of a body that is a measure of its inertia, that is commonly taken as a measure of the amount of material it contains and causes it to have weight in a gravitational field, and that along with length and time constitutes one of the fundamental quantities on which all physical measurements are based."

What that means is that the mass of a planet has a lot to do with the weight of an object on that planet. Jupiter's mass is 318 times that of Earth, therefore, the force of gravity on Jupiter is much greater than that on Earth. For example, a one hundred pound object on Earth would weigh about 240 pounds on Jupiter. Everything would be a lot heavier on Jupiter, again relating to our study of weight.

But although Jupiter has a large mass, it has a low density. Density is defined as the mass of a substance per unit volume, again per Webster. The density of Jupiter is slightly more than that of water, and it is about a fourth as dense as the Earth. So, instead of being solid like Earth, Jupiter is just a big ball of gas (about 90% hydrogen and 10% helium). It would be impossible for a spacecraft to land there. In other words, Jupiter is large but it is expansive. It carries a lot of mass, but it is lightweight mass.

Like the planet Saturn, Jupiter too has rings, but they are not nearly as large as Saturn's rings and they are somewhat thin and faint. The rings, which are closer to Jupiter than any of its satellites, are believed by scientists to be composed of rock fragments.

The outer edges of the rings are very sharply defined, but the inner edges are somewhat fuzzy. A thin sheet of material from the rings extends from the inner edge all the way down to the planet's upper atmosphere.

Jupiter has satellites that rotate around it, four of them large enough to qualify as moons, and the rest just small bodies that follow it around. William J. Kaufmann in the book, *Universe*, says that the densities of the four moons decrease as the distance from Jupiter increases, which mimics the solar system. He goes on to say that as you move outward from the Sun, the average density of the planets steadily decreases. Scientists therefore believe that Jupiter's moons were formed in a process much like the process that formed our solar system, albeit it on a smaller scale.

Jupiter is a very colorful planet of reds, oranges, browns, and yellows. When you look at it through a telescope, you see a series of alternating dark and light areas, or belts and zones. The belts are dark colored lines, and the zones are lighter colored areas. Scientists speculate that these belts and zones are probably caused by the differing temperatures of the various gases in the clouds. Jupiter emits more heat than it receives from the Sun. The clouds are believed to vary in temperature and therefore to vary in depth in Jupiter's atmosphere. Brown clouds are thought to be the warmest and so make up the deepest layers. Whitish clouds, and then red clouds, form the next highest layers respectively. In addition to the belts and zones, Jupiter has a large, red-orange oval called the Great Red Spot.

Jupiter takes about twelve years (eleven years and 314 days to be exact) to revolve around the Sun.

THE GLYPH FOR JUPITER

There are three basic symbols that combine in different ways to form the symbols or glyphs for the planets. In other words, the glyphs for the planets each have unique meanings based upon the placement and relationship of these three symbols. The three symbols are the circle, the crescent and the cross. The circle represents spirit, or the eternal, the crescent represents the personality, and the cross represents earth, or matter.

The glyph for Jupiter utilizes two of the three symbols, the crescent and the cross. It looks like the number four. It represents the personality rising above the earth or matter. The significance of the glyph is that nothing earthly can restrict or confine the personality. Another way of saying this is that even though we live in a material world, the inner or spiritual side of our nature is in control, thereby lifting the personality to a higher level. Astrologers often use the term "consciousness raising" when referring to Jupiter transits.

WHAT JUPITER'S NAME MEANS

Next, let's look at Jupiter's namesake, the mighty Roman god. Astrologers often look at the mythological meanings of the names of the various planets, hoping to gain additional insight into their astrological significance. There is a school of thought which espouses the belief that the names of the planets are not coincidental; that the names are chosen because of a sub-conscious connection to the universal mind. This same school of thought also feels that the entire mythological lore has its basis in universal principles, and so it is quite appropriate to assign characteristics of a particular mythological figure to the planet bearing its name. Whether or not you agree with these theories, the similarities between the mythological and astrological qualities of the various planets is incontrovertible.

In Roman mythology, Jupiter was the king of the gods and the ruler of the universe. He was known as Zeus in Greek mythology. Jupiter was the god of celestial light. He was also the god of thunder and is many times depicted with thunderbolts.

Jupiter was the son of Saturn (Cronus in Greek mythology), the reigning god of the universe. But Jupiter and his siblings dethroned Saturn in an interesting tale. The story has it that Saturn, having been warned that one day one of his children would dethrone him, decided that the best way to avoid this undesired happening was to swallow his children as soon as they were born. Saturn's wife was tired of this behavior, so the next time she gave birth, instead of handing the baby to Saturn, she handed him a large stone wrapped in baby clothes. Saturn swallowed the stone, and thus Jupiter's life was saved. After years of fighting, Jupiter eventually won and claimed the throne.

Jupiter was married to the goddess Juno (Hera in Greek mythology). They had a stormy marriage, and he had many mistresses and illegitimate children. Jupiter was well aware of Juno's jealousy, as she often took revenge on his lovers. In spite of the threat of Juno's retaliation, Jupiter continually and enthusiastically pursued goddesses and mortal women alike throughout the course of their marriage. He was forever taking different forms, such as eagles, cuckoos, pigeons, swans and bulls in order to seduce his amorous interests. Once he even became a shower of gold so that he could enter a tower in which Danae, one of his love interests, had been locked. He was quite ingenious and persistent when it came to satisfying his passion for affairs of the heart.

In spite of these infidelities, Jupiter was still considered a wise sovereign, believed to be basically fair in his dispensation of good and evil. He was, for the most part, presented as being kind and compassionate, and a defender of the weak.

TRADITIONAL ASTROLOGICAL
INTERPRETATION OF JUPITER

Now that you know a little something about Jupiter's namesake and its glyph, it should be pretty easy to understand the traditional meaning of Jupiter. Jupiter is the planet of luck, opportunity and expansion. Wherever you find Jupiter in your chart is where you will be fortunate, as it represents material, intellectual, and spiritual success. Jupiter denotes optimism, so that you will always see the positive side of every situation. The principle of expansion is powerful with this planet, and the result is that Jupiter shows a desire to expand your knowledge, explore your world, and broaden your point of view.

Jupiter has a very spiritual connotation, and has to do with your philosophical, moral or spiritual point of view and values. The placement of Jupiter in your chart indicates your level of spiritual development and the direction of the development and growth of your soul in this life. You find your spiritual purpose with Jupiter. It is the planet that rules kindness, charity, benevolence, and friendship.

Jupiter is big—big in all the wonderful qualities and feelings that humanity appreciates: joy, happiness, prosperity, wealth, optimism, inspiration, warmth, love, compassion, wisdom, friendliness, hope, rewards, personal power and spiritual purpose. He is the Santa Claus of the universe.

JUPITER: A FAILED SUN?

We have already discussed the fact that Jupiter's chemical composition is about 90% hydrogen and 10% helium. This chemical composition is very similar to that of the Sun. We also discussed earlier that scientists believe that the same processes that formed our solar system formed the moons of Jupiter.

Scientists have long theorized that had Jupiter been larger, it would have collapsed to form a star. Nancy Hathaway, in *The Friendly Guide to the Universe*, says that if some cosmic mason were to pack extra matter around it [Jupiter], the effort would only compress the planet, causing it to shrink. If however, enough matter were added to equal seventy to eighty times Jupiter's actual mass, the rising temperature and internal pressure would spark nuclear reactions, and Jupiter would no longer be a planet, but would become a star, which means that it would produce heat. Indeed, its core is hotter than the surface of the Sun, and it generates nearly twice as much heat as it receives from the Sun.

So is Jupiter a failed star? That's something to ponder.

LARGE VS. LIGHT

Now that we know quite a bit about Jupiter, let's see if we can make sense of all this information. What can we say is the hidden meaning, the significance, of Jupiter? Let's come up with some key words for Jupiter based upon what we have learned and maybe by putting them all together, we can arrive at the true nature and function of this large planet. Let's start with the word large. Large, enormous, and yet lightweight. These we learn from Jupiter's physical description. From its mythological namesake, we learn that he is quite powerful, too, or at least he emits quite a bit of heat. We weigh more on Jupiter than we do on Earth. From Jupiter's mythological namesake, we can glean the words power, might, kindness and compassion as he doled out punishments and rewards in a fair and just manner. The fact that the mythological god would not allow himself to be confined or limited to only one woman again emphasizes the quality of expansiveness. And from traditional astrology, we learn the words light and enlightener, expansiveness, openness, optimism, love, faith, and spiritualism. Finally, from the glyph for Jupiter, we learn that he has been given the role of lifting or raising our personality to a higher level.

Could it be, then, that the significance of Jupiter is to allow for the expansion of our consciousness in a large and yet light or lightweight way? That he seeks to broaden our ability to love in an open and flexible manner? And could it be that excess weight, from Jupiter's perspective, represents either our refusal or inability to successfully expand or enlighten our consciousness? Do we become large in the physical sense because we did not become large when asked by Jupiter in the spiritual sense? Is excess weight just the visible manifestation of an aborted attempt at an expansion of consciousness? Could it be that when Jupiter comes to us and asks that we raise our consciousness to a new level, that we expand and grow philosophically, morally, or spiritually and we refuse, we punish ourselves by carrying around that failed experience as excess weight? Could it be that if we do in fact allow the consciousness expansion to occur, that the excess weight becomes "light" or "lightweight" or "enlightenment?"

Hold that thought.

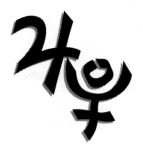

CHAPTER TWO

UNDERSTANDING PLUTO, THE ELIMINATOR

Now we are going to take a look at a planet that is pretty much the opposite of Jupiter. Pluto is small, dark, and secretive, as opposed to Jupiter's largesse, colorful presentation and expansiveness. And yet, Pluto is just as powerful as his brother. Take a look.

PLUTO, THE SMALLEST PLANET

Pluto is the smallest, coldest and probably the strangest of all the planets. Pluto is slightly smaller than our moon. Pluto is a shiny, frozen world, made of rock and various kinds of reflective ice. The planet's surface is covered with icy methane, nitrogen and carbon monoxide, and its thin atmosphere is comprised of these same elements. Scientists believe that Pluto's tenuous atmosphere has a pressure perhaps only a few millionths of that at the surface of the Earth, and a person on Pluto would weigh quite a bit less than they weigh on Earth.

Most of the time, Pluto is the farthest planet from the Sun, and is about 39 times as far from the Sun as the Earth is. Pluto takes 6.39 days to rotate on its axis, which it does on its side. It takes the planet about 248 years to revolve around the Sun. It is not always the farthest planet from the Sun, though, for its orbit is extremely elongated and it varies between 4,400 and 7,400 million kilometers from the Sun. Its orbit is wildly eccentric and extremely tilted and elliptical. In fact, it is so much more elliptical than other planetary orbits that at one point in its journey, Pluto crosses over the orbit of Neptune, bringing it inside Neptune's orbit, which then makes Neptune the most distant planet. Pluto remains inside Neptune's orbit for about twenty years.

Pluto has one moon, Charon, named after the mythological boatman who ferried souls across the River Styx to Hades, the underground world ruled by Pluto. Charon is slightly over half the size of Pluto, which makes it the largest moon in the solar system in relation to the planet around which it revolves.

We don't know as much about Pluto as we do about the other planets in our solar system because Pluto is the only planet that has not yet been visited by a spacecraft.

THE GLYPH FOR PLUTO

The glyph for Pluto is made up of all three symbols, that is, the circle, the crescent, and the cross. Remember from the discussion of Jupiter in Chapter One, that the circle represents spirit or the eternal, the crescent represents the personality, and the cross represents the earth, or matter.

In the glyph for Pluto, the crescent is above the cross, and the circle is above them both. Not only has the personality ascended the earth or matter, but it has also connected with spirit, or the eternal. In other words, through Pluto, the eternal spirit descends into matter and the result is an ascended personality or soul consciousness. The symbol seems to be saying that the purpose of Pluto is to aid in the development of this soul consciousness.

WHAT PLUTO'S NAME MEANS

In Roman mythology, Pluto is the god of the dead, the god of the underworld. (He is called Hades in Greek mythology.) Pluto is Jupiter's brother, and at the time that Jupiter took control of the world after defeating their father, Saturn, Jupiter divided the various parts of the world between himself and his brothers, Pluto and Neptune. Neptune was given control of the seas, and Pluto was given control of the underworld.

The name Pluto means "riches" and it is true that Pluto rules buried treasures, so to speak. Pluto rules over the underworld and he rules over it absolutely. And he seems quite content to be there, having only left his kingdom two times, once to abduct his wife Proserpina (or Persephone in Greek mythology), and the other time to go in search of a cure for a wound to his shoulder inflicted by Hercules.

The story of how Pluto abducted his wife is quite dramatic. One day while Proserpina was in a field gathering flowers with her companions, she noticed a beautiful narcissus. As she bent down to pick the flower, the earth opened up and Pluto arose from the chasm, surprising Proserpina. He carried her away in his chariot and plunged with her into the depths of the earth. Her mother, Ceres (Demeter in Greek mythology), who was the goddess of vegetation and fruitfulness, was quite devastated, and refused to allow anything to grow on Earth until her daughter was returned to her. Jupiter finally had to intervene, and to make a long story short, Proserpina was ordered to live six months of the year with her mother, Ceres on Earth, and six months in the underworld with her husband, Pluto.

If Pluto ever did choose to leave the underworld and visit Earth, he had one special trick. He could visit the world above and not be seen for his helmet made him invisible.

As far as fidelity in marriage was concerned, Pluto was much more faithful to Proserpine than Jupiter was to Juno. There were only two occasions noted where Pluto was unfaithful to his wife.

TRADITIONAL ASTROLOGICAL
INTREPRETATION OF PLUTO

The astrological significance of the planet Pluto is death, transformation and rebirth. Symbolically, Pluto's effect is like a volcano; it seethes and bubbles under the surface, until one day it finally explodes, and after the smoke and ash have subsided, the old landscape is totally demolished, and is ready for a whole new look.

Pluto encourages you to give something up, but replaces it with something better. That is why it is called the planet of elimination and death. It assists you in eliminating whatever is blocking your progress, so that a new and improved version of yourself can emerge. Pluto does this with laser beam accuracy and efficiency. Pluto's transformations are dramatic and permanent. Pluto's transits can seem very harsh, brutal, and drastic, and if we fight them, then Pluto transits can be very hard to endure. You can literally feel as if you are in hell.

Pluto symbolizes the idea of making sure we fulfill our spiritual destiny. Pluto's placement in your natal chart shows you where you need to make the largest transformation in your life because it is the area that is keeping you from achieving your soul's purpose.

So far, it sounds like Pluto's significance is totally negative, but that is certainly not the case. Pluto symbolizes willpower, inner strength, stamina, and resourcefulness. With a powerful and positive Pluto in your chart, you can strategize and almost always reach your goal. If you work with the energies represented by Pluto instead of fighting them, you can make major progress in transforming your personality.

And let's not forget that Pluto also symbolizes intensity of emotion. Pluto often signifies a strong sex drive, but that is only one manifestation of the passion that this planet represents. A strong Pluto in your chart indicates that you are emotionally passionate about everything, not just sex.

Pluto is also linked to secrecy, to the dark or hidden side of things. Pluto goes down to the underworld or the hidden areas of our lives, and brings up all the dirt and muck so that it can be eliminated. If you have any skeletons in your closet, and we all do, prepare to have them surface when Pluto transits that area of your life.

The words, then, that most aptly describe the symbolic significance of Pluto would be death, transformation, elimination, intensity, power and passion.

THE LITTLE PLANET WITH THE BIG MOON

So what can we conclude about the littlest planet? What is its purpose, its significance? From the discussion of its physical characteristics, we learn that it is small, dark, mysterious, and cold. It is powerful, too, for it controls a moon that is over half its size.

The word elimination also applies, since we weigh less on Pluto than on Earth. From its mythological namesake, we see again most of those same qualities. Pluto represents death and darkness for he lives under the Earth. He is secretive because he is able to roam the Earth unseen with his invisible helmet, and he is quite powerful as he is the absolute ruler of the underworld. And from his astrological meaning, we again see the words death, elimination and transformation. Finally, the glyph for Pluto indicates that he has been allotted the task of seeing to it that we align ourselves with our spiritual purpose.

In Pluto's case, then, can we conclude that he performs his symbolic function of aligning us with our spiritual purpose by ridding us of or eliminating anything that is not in line with that purpose? Could it be that if we allow this death, elimination and the resulting transformation to take place, that physically, or ostensibly, this "elimination" manifests as a loss of weight? And could it be that if we refuse to allow this death, elimination and transformational process to take place, the failed effort remains with us ostensibly as excess weight?

Let's explore those ideas in detail in the next chapters.

"That's all well and good," sighed the princess, after sitting patiently through three hours of lecturing by the little elf, "but, Sebastian, how is that information going to help me shed my extra weight?"

Sebastian took his time in answering. Sebastian did everything slowly and deliberately, too slowly sometimes for the princess' tastes. Finally, he bent down and picked a beautiful, healthy yellow wildflower close to the rock upon which the princess was sitting.

"Study this flower," he said, as he handed it to the princess. "It began as a beautiful thought. Then this beautiful thought received all the proper nutrients, and plenty of sunlight and water, and has responded by blooming into this most magnificent flower. It is the best that it can be. It is the beautiful thought made tangible." Then he bent down and picked another wildflower, only this one was rather sickly looking, having grown in the shade so it had not received the proper amount of sunlight or water in order to bloom properly.

"*Compare this sickly flower to the beautiful specimen you hold in your hand. It...*"

Before he could finish, the princess interrupted him.

"*Are you comparing me to this sickly flower? Do you think there's something sick about me because I weigh a few extra pounds?*" *she asked belligerently.*

"*Absolutely not!*" *he exclaimed.* "*But maybe there were certain nutrients that you needed and either you could not or did not receive them, and so maybe you didn't develop quite the way you should have. But you are like the sick flower which only needs a little loving care, the right nutrients, and plenty of water and sunshine, and it can turn into a flower as beautiful as the first.*"

The princess was now totally confused, for she did not know if she should be angry with the little elf or if she should hug him. The elf, sensing her dilemma, suggested that this might be a good time to take a break. She agreed, and so the two of them set out on a leisurely walk along the river's edge. The princess was beginning to have her doubts about the wisdom of this little elf, and needed some time to think. What was he trying to tell her exactly, and did it really make any sense, she asked herself.

They walked in silence and after about ten minutes, came upon a large grove of apple trees. The princess immediately picked one for herself.

"*Care for an apple?*" *she asked Sebastian.* "*I'll pick one for you, if you'd like.*" *Since Sebastian was only two feet tall and therefore could not reach even the lowest branch, she naively assumed that he would appreciate her offer.*

"*Put me on your shoulders and I'll pick my own, thank you.*"

The princess obeyed. She bent down, and Sebastian deftly placed himself on her shoulders, so that when she stood up, he was in perfect position to reach even the highest branches. Sebastian, as it turned out, was extremely discriminating when it came to apples, so it took him a while to find just the right one. But the princess knew that his patience had been rewarded as soon as she saw his choice. After gently returning Sebastian to the ground, she observed with great interest the fruit in the elf's little blue hand. It was perfectly round and red. But more importantly, it seemed to have a quality that none of the other apples had. It had the most beautiful sheen that she had ever seen on an apple. As a matter of fact, it seemed to be the shiniest of all the apples on the tree.

The princess and Sebastian sat on the ground beside the river and ate their apples in silence. Hers was sweet and juicy, with just enough crunch to make it exciting, but she knew that it was not nearly as sweet, juicy nor as crunchy as Sebastian's, judging by the look of contentment on his face. When they finished their fruit, they tossed the cores into the river. Two large, magenta birds with golden tipped wings gracefully glided down from a nearby tree and grabbed them just seconds before they would have hit the water. It was a thrilling sight. Finally Sebastian spoke.

"I think we should continue your lessons now."

The princess looked worried. Even after their little respite, she was still wrestling with the discussion they had had about the flowers. So before allowing the lessons to proceed, she knew she had to summon the courage to ask him the question that was weighing heavily on her mind.

"Do you really think that there is hope for me?" asked the princess.

"Most assuredly," Sebastian replied.

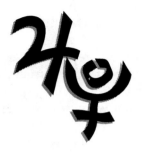

CHAPTER THREE
THE BASIC ASTROLOGICAL RULES
OF WEIGHT CONTROL

Rule Number One: If Jupiter is trying to enlighten us, and we refuse to be enlightened, that unfulfilled idea or unrealized thought stays with us and manifests in the physical world as excess weight.

Rule Number Two: If Pluto is asking us to eliminate something from our lives and we refuse, that unfulfilled idea or unrealized thought stays with us and manifests in the physical world as excess weight.

Rule Number Three: All change is positive and should be embraced.

These three rules are the essence of astrological weight control. If you want to lose weight, it is merely a matter of analyzing your life to determine where it is that Jupiter has been trying to enlighten you, or what it is that Pluto wants you to eliminate, and then just make the change. Simple, right?

The largest planet and the smallest planet each have their own agendas, and their own methods of operation. Both methods are extremely effective for they are both able to get our attention. Of the two types of energy symbolized by these two planets, Jupiter's is the more palatable, and therefore probably the easier to deal with. Jupiter is indicative of energy that is usually regarded positively, i.e., it represents generous, benevolent and optimistic feelings so, in most cases, we look forward to Jupiter's visits to our chart. Plutonian energy, on the other hand, can sometimes seem very negative and even dreary at times. Where Jovian energy represents feelings of joy, Plutonian energy can sometimes depict very sinister and dark feelings. This is because Pluto symbolizes feelings and areas of our lives that are very low, things that we would prefer to keep hidden.

When these two planets show up in our horoscope, we usually know what they want, even if we say we don't. When they come knocking with their particular cosmic message, we have probably had an inkling of what this whole thing is going to be all about long before they actually make themselves known. If we say that we don't—that we were totally surprised—we are really saying that we are not connected to our inner self, for the subconscious always knows.

But for argument's sake, let's assume that we do not know what these planets are asking from us. If you want to figure out what they want, think back to the last time you experienced an unwelcome weight gain. What was going on in your life at that time? If the weight gain was Jupiter-related, you need to look for areas of your life where you were being short-sighted, where a broader perspective might have helped. Look for issues of enlightenment that deal with new ideas, new ways of doing things or approaching problems, or new ways of thinking. The word "enlighten" is defined as giving intellectual or spiritual light, as instructing or imparting knowledge, or to shed light upon something. What Jupiter is symbolically attempting to do is to remove you from your old mindset, and show you a whole new way of seeing the world. Jupiter is indicative of energy that takes you from your narrow perspective to a larger, more inclusive one. With Jupiter, you never really lose what you already know—you just expand upon it.

And yet there are many who fear the mind-expanding efforts implied by Jupiter because they are afraid of what lies ahead. They know what the present is all about, and even if that present is painfully limiting, they fear change because they don't know what it will bring. Jupiter's symbolic goal is to take you to larger and larger, all-inclusive, spheres of experience. Therefore, this experience is nothing to be frightened of. To repeat, you are not losing anything. When you learn to look at the world in a different, more inclusive way, you lose nothing and you gain perspective.

Those of us who are more flexible have a much easier time with this transition than those who are not, and this is a subject I will deal with in depth in the next chapter. But for now, it is important to understand that we can all do this. We can all expand our knowledge and learn to see the world in a different way, if we only allow ourselves to do so. We need to give ourselves permission to be fearless, to dare to believe that there may be a different way of doing things, a better, more inclusive way. To accept Jupiter's symbolic gift of enlightenment, and it is definitely a gift, we need to allow it to happen without fighting it. That requires giving up a certain amount of control, and some of us are not comfortable doing that. However, we can learn to do it, especially if we don't try to do it all at once. All we need to do is to start out with small steps, baby steps, and gradually we will arrive at our destination.

Pluto's goal is a little different, and may require a little more effort on our part. While becoming enlightened under Jupiter's watch merely requires that we allow it to happen, in order for Pluto to succeed, we must consciously give up something. And if we are extremely attached to that which he is asking us to give up, then Pluto's visit may be a very painful and difficult experience. In this elimination process, the only way to make it painless is to lose the strong desire we have for the item that is being eliminated. This thing that Pluto is asking us to give up may be as simple as an ill-conceived idea, or as important as a marriage partner, our home, or our way of life.

If you are struggling with the elimination process indicative of Plutonian energy, it might help to tell yourself over and over that you are being asked to give something up so that you can receive something better in its place. Remembering that fact should take the scariness out of relinquishing the known for the unknown. If the unknown is better, then it can't be bad, right? The other trick is to try to relax and use the same approach suggested for a

Jupiter enlightenment process, namely, just allow it to happen. Don't fight it. In most cases, you will be happy to see that situation or that person or whatever you are being asked to give up, leave your life. It's probably been a big hassle anyway, so you should be ready for some relief and a change for the better. People always want to hang onto what is familiar in their lives, even though it may be the worst for them. Let it go. Once you clear out the old mess, new, wonderful things can come in.

If you are fighting against it, the energy represented by Pluto can sometimes result in feelings that are very depressing and heavy. However, once you allow the transformation suggested by Pluto, you will find that you are blessed with a sense of total freedom, and that heavy burdens have been lifted. Clearing out the clutter in our lives (and clutter can be unhappy relationships, debt issues, etc.) can make us feel new again. Astrologers often use the word transformation when referring to Pluto transits, because this process of elimination does allow you to transform yourself into that new person who was waiting behind the scenes. Transformation always requires getting rid of the old so that the new can emerge.

In dealing with both of these energies, then, the secret is to just let it happen. Be open to change. After all, that's what life is all about. We're here to learn and grow, and if we fight it, we are only hurting ourselves. Carrying around unnecessary baggage can weigh us down mentally, emotionally and physically so the smartest thing to do is to let it go. And as you do, you will see the weight leave also. Fighting enlightenment can be damaging to your body mentally, emotionally and physically also. Allow yourself to be enlightened and you will see the weight "lighten up" and disappear.

And how do you just allow change to happen? This brings us to rule number three. If you are able to view all change in a positive light, then you are well on your way to permanent weight control. Unfortunately, many people have difficulty in viewing change positively for a variety of reasons, and the next chapter looks at some of them.

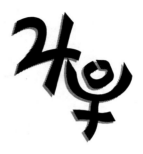

CHAPTER FOUR

THE ROLE OF THE PSYCHE IN WEIGHT CONTROL

The way in which you perceive reality has a lot to do with the sign on your Ascendant. This is because your Ascendant represents your psyche or soul. Your moon sign represents your past, especially your emotional and biological past, and your sun sign is your current personality, but your Ascendant is what you are ascending or aspiring to be. It represents your soul characteristics. The dictionary defines psyche as the human soul, spirit, or mind, or the mental or psychological structure of a person. This psychological structure, therefore, greatly influences how the psyche, or soul, perceives its reality. How your psyche perceives reality is important because it has a bearing on how you react to it.

The nature of your psyche or soul is important to us in our study of weight because success in interpreting and correctly responding to Jupiter and Pluto motifs is directly related to how you perceive reality. Since the way you perceive reality has a direct bearing on whether or not you make correct assessments and decisions, it follows that your perception of reality directly affects your mental, emotional and physical weight. To properly analyze Jupiter and Pluto drives requires flexibility and a large amount of optimism and trust in the universe and in the future. Certain Ascendants are more flexible and trusting and therefore have an easier time expanding their consciousness, or releasing unnecessary burdens. They are able to instinctively rely on the goodness and wisdom of the universe. They understand that there is a master plan and that everything proceeds according to the natural laws of the universe, and that everything works out for the best possible good. These Ascendants normally have no problem, then, in accepting change because they know how to flow with the natural currents of the universe.

We normally label this ability to flow with changes as flexibility. When it comes to flexibility, the mutable signs, Gemini, Virgo, Sagittarius and Pisces, are the most flexible, and therefore would have the easiest time adjusting to changes required by Jupiter or Pluto. It follows logically that those signs that would have the most difficulty in adjusting to change would be the fixed signs, namely, Taurus, Leo, Scorpio, and Aquarius. And falling somewhere in the middle would be the cardinal signs of Aries, Cancer, Libra and Capricorn.

Having an Ascendant in one of the fixed signs, then, would make it more difficult to assimilate change, because it would make the psyche view situations more pessimistically, and therefore not see the opportunities inherent in transformational situations. If one's Ascendant is in one of the fixed signs, change is viewed as something bad, something to be avoided at all costs. Why this is so varies with each of the four fixed signs, and I will try to explain these differences in detail in the discussion of the various Ascendants at the end of this chapter.

Because we create our own reality based on our perceptions, it follows that if we interpret situations in a positive manner, our lives will turn out positively. Here's an example.

Two women, the same age, both have their only child leaving home for the first time to enter college. Mom number one sees this as a negative. She is losing her baby, she is dreading the empty nest syndrome, she is worried that she won't be there if her child needs her, and as a result, she eats more, gains weight, and can't understand her depression. Mom number two sees her child leaving as a testament to her great mothering skills. Feeling that she has done a successful job in the motherhood arena, she is anxious to see what life has next in store for her. She feels energized; takes up jogging, and loses ten pounds.

The same situation is perceived in two entirely different ways, producing opposite results. Our perception of reality conditions our reactions, which in turn creates our reality. It is a never-ending cycle. So before we can start applying the rules of astrological weight loss, we need to take a look at our Ascendant, our perceiving apparatus, and determine if we need to do some work in that area. Every opportunity that we are given to change is a chance for us to learn and grow; if we do not perceive change in that way, we are limiting ourselves, holding ourselves back, and carrying around that limitation in the form of excess weight. Now, take a look at your Ascendant in the following table, and see if you need to do some work on your perceptions. In the discussion of each of the Ascendants, I analyze the traits of the opposite sign as a tool to learn how to change your mode of perception. The sign opposite your Ascendant possesses traits that you are lacking, and in order to become well rounded, some of these missing traits need to be fused with your Ascendant sign traits.

ARIES ASCENDANT

A person with an Aries Ascendant perceives reality solely as it affects him or herself personally. Therefore, if no connection can be made between the required change and personal benefit, it will be disregarded. If a benefit can be seen, the Aries rising person will immediately agree to make the change, without a second thought. With this rising sign, everything is done hastily, with not too much attention paid to details. They are not afraid to act and will jump right in. So the issue for anyone with this rising sign is to avoid the tendency to hastily dismiss the benefits of a suggested Jupiterian or Plutonian change. "Slow down" might be their code words. They need to stop and ask themselves what the benefit of responding to this request might be. They must dig a little deeper.

One way to do this, Aries, is to look to the traits of the opposite sign, which in this case is Libra. Librans are noted for their ability to weigh all the facts before making a decision. You don't necessarily have to carry it to extremes, for sometimes Librans can become so weighted down with facts that they cannot make a decision. All you need to do is to learn to look a little more at the pros and cons of the issue, and with your Aries-quick mentality you will be able to make a correct decision; one based on the correct facts. With all the facts, you will realize that all change is necessary, and that all change brings benefits. You will recognize those benefits and will then be able to charge forward, which is your usual manner.

TAURUS ASCENDANT

This is the first of the fixed signs, and so an Ascendant found here would be very averse to change, and would perceive change as something to be stopped, or held at bay. For a Taurus rising person, anything that stands in the way of its goal is suspect, and unless the person is very advanced, and can properly see the goal, he will misinterpret the nature of the change and see it as a road-block. The great thing about Taurus rising individuals is that they are committed to achieving their goal. So the issue for them would be to make sure they correctly perceive the goal.

Again, taking a look at the traits of the opposite sign, Scorpio, would shed some light on how to overcome this perception issue. How can Scorpio traits help you see change as being a positive event? The sign of Scorpio is where we are tested; it is where we are presented with major crises and then are required to confront our problem areas and defeat them. Adopting a Scorpionic willingness to confront our demons and slay them can challenge your stubbornness and tenacity. If you approached change with the perspective that you have the strength and resourcefulness to vanquish your weaknesses, clearing your path to higher goals and aspirations, your perception of change would become positive. Your mindset would shift from one of avoiding change at all costs to one of relishing change, for it affords the opportunity to slay your demons and move on to what you really want to do.

GEMINI ASCENDANT

Gemini energy is scattered all over the place; trying anything different, novel, or unusual. Thus, it is not only easy for a Gemini rising person to change, but it is something they look forward to. Gemini is the first of the mutable signs, and so is by definition, extremely flexible. Perception of change by those with Gemini Ascendants is normally one of acceptance, excitement and adventure. Admittedly, if one has strong earth influence in one's chart, even having a Gemini Ascendant may not be enough to make you feel comfortable with change, but at least your perception of it will be positive, and this will allow you to make a smoother transition.

One of your positive characteristics, Gemini rising, is your ability to relish change. However, it can also be your downfall. Change is good, but you must spend enough time living with a particular change to understand why it was necessary. If, in your zest to experience more and more new things, you miss the point of the current change, you may end up spending your lives chasing one thing after another, and the true value of the experience will have been lost. You can learn how to avoid this by looking to your opposite sign, Sagittarius, and incorporating the archer's balancing act. Before shooting his arrow, the Sagittarian takes time to balance himself, to make sure that his stance is solid, and then he moves on. You need to incorporate the idea of pausing to reflect upon the nature of the change, to incorporate it fully in to your life—to "balance" yourself, so to speak, before moving on to the next experience.

CANCER ASCENDANT

Cancer rising's perception of reality is usually tinged with a sense of trepidation, and as a result, change is an unwanted commodity. Because the home and foundation are so important to those with this rising sign, change is perceived as something that will erode their base, their safe harbor. Those with Cancer rising have the opportunity to be a beacon for others searching for some sort of foundation in their lives; the Cancer rising individual can be an example, but only if he or she chooses to take a detached rather than personal view of the environment. Once they have developed this attitude of detachment, Cancer rising individuals can decipher rather easily the cries for help of the masses, and as the mother or nurturer of the zodiac, can provide aid and comfort to many.

This necessary detachment to fulfill the mothering role to the masses can be learned once again, by paying attention to the traits of your opposite sign, Capricorn. Capricorn is known for its ability to remain detached, and to do whatever is necessary without allowing emotions to get in the way. If you are facing change, rather than immediately reacting to the change in a emotional way, that is, seeing the change as a threat to your security, you should instead endeavor to view it rationally and unemotionally, as an ambitious opportunity to expand your base, foundation, home, etc. Change can then be perceived as an opening to a higher level of existence, a step up in status and an instrument to make a beneficial contribution to a larger and more inclusive world.

LEO ASCENDANT

The main perception problem of those born with the regal Leo Ascendant is the perception that everything revolves around you and your needs, so any change that you did not request is of no interest to you. Leo rising people have a very highly developed sense of self, and while there is nothing wrong with this, it can create a feeling of self-satisfaction and impede further growth. Leo is one of the fixed signs, and is so confident in its own abilities to assess a situation, that many times, the Leo rising person will not even entertain the ideas and opinions of others. Change, if initiated by others is simply dismissed.

To correct this perception of change, you should study the traits of your opposite sign, Aquarius. Aquarius is the sign of the humanitarian, the person with the universal point of view. Aquarius individuals understand that we are all connected, and that everything that affects one of us affects all of us. If you were to color your perception of change with this idea of a universal rather than a self-centered view of change, you would then be able to allow for the idea of being part of a larger, more inclusive purpose, and therefore, be more amenable to the change. Understanding that change will benefit the larger whole, will, in most cases, stimulate that large Leo heart of yours into embracing the change for the good of all.

VIRGO ASCENDANT

Virgo is another of the mutable signs, and so someone with this Ascendant should have very little problem perceiving change as positive. However, there can be a downside to this rising sign's assessment of change, and that is that one can become so discriminating and so exacting, that he or she may miss out on some important opportunities for soul growth. Virgo rising people can be the snobs of the zodiac. It is fine to want the best, but sometimes they may not recognize the best because they are too quick to dismiss anything that they don't understand. They need to make an effort to understand points of view different from their own or those not like themselves.

Looking to your opposite sign of Pisces can help you tremendously in that area. Pisces is the sign of compassion, and is able to actually feel the pain of others. It can look into the hearts of strangers and know what is there. While it is not necessary for you to become as compassionate and feeling as the person with Pisces rising, if you want to better assimilate change, you need to become more sensitive and open to the plight of others, which will then allow you to better interpret situations requiring change of some sort. You will then be able to see the benefits of the change more clearly, and then can apply your Virgoan ability to perceive it as positive. By allowing yourself to be a little less quick to judge, by looking at all situations from a position of compassion and understanding, you will be able to spot more opportunities for personal change and growth. By only looking for change that is absolutely perfect, you miss a lot of worthwhile opportunities, because not everything worthwhile is perfectly arranged or perfectly presented.

LIBRA ASCENDANT

The Libra rising person is most concerned with balance. Everything must be harmonious, as discord upsets this person physically, mentally and emotionally. Those with Libran Ascendants are celebrated for their impartiality and their ability to view both sides of any issue before making a decision. Their final decision is one that, at least in their minds, is just and right.

Therefore, if a person with Libra rising perceives change in a negative light, it is probably related to the fact that the changes are somehow throwing their world out of kilter, out of harmony. Having looked at the pros and cons of making the change, the Libran rising native has come to the conclusion that the change will do more harm than good, or that the benefits of staying where he is outweigh those of changing.

Sometimes, also, a Libran Ascendant will choose not to make a change because he or she is overwhelmed with information and cannot sift through it to make a decision, and therefore makes no decision. In this case, the Libra Ascendant person will sit on the fence forever, until someone or something comes along to knock him off, which is the worst possible of all endings. Having the decision made for a Libra rising person does not allow him any input, and this could be totally contrary to his wishes or best interests.

So how do you learn to embrace change if you have a Libra Ascendant? Again, by looking to the traits of the opposite sign, Aries. A person with an Aries Ascendant acts on his instincts. He does not need mountains of evidence to support his actions. If he feels it is right, he does it. Aries is the pioneer, and the way you become a pioneer is to be the first, to just step out there and do it. Emulating Aries, you need to develop the ability to recognize when something just feels right for you and then do it. You need to understand that sometimes you don't need facts, or evidence, or even logic—when something feels right, you have permission to toss out the scales. So what if things are out of whack temporarily? You will eventually get back in balance, and regaining that balance is part of the learning and growth process. Viewing change as positive allows you to rid yourself of that awful feeling of not being able to make a decision.

SCORPIO ASCENDANT

Those with Scorpio Ascendants are very strong-willed people indeed. They are secretive, resourceful and resilient. They have a tendency to see everything as a battle, and everyone as an enemy, so change is normally perceived by these people as something not to be trusted, but instead as something to be defeated or over-come. They will strategize and use their scorpionic inner strength to fight off change for as long as possible, until the death, in some instances, which can really limit their opportunities for soul growth. Being resourceful and possessing a strong will are excellent traits and can be very useful as one journeys through life. However, since life is about growth, these scorpionic traits need to be adjusted so that they are useful in that arena.

By looking at the opposite sign, Taurus, you can learn to make an adjustment in your perception of change by adopting the Taurean quality of striving towards a goal. If you do that, you will eventually come to the realization that change is necessary if one is to arrive at the desired goal. Whatever one aspires to do, there must be a path to follow in order to get there and it is quite logical to believe that change is not bad if it will assist us in arriving at the goal. To desire, or aspire, requires that certain steps be taken and changes be assimilated. By accepting this point of view, you can begin to understand the value of change, and can then better assess what to fight and what not to fight. By accepting the notion that change can be beneficial to achieve your goal, you can begin to perceive change as an opportunity to use your warrior skills in a positive, beneficial way which will aid in your soul growth.

SAGITTARIUS ASCENDANT

A Sagittarius rising person perceives change, for the most part, as positive, since this is one of the mutable signs. But sometimes a Sagittarius rising person has problems in this area because they are oftentimes too dogmatic in their views, and as a result, if an opportunity for change presents itself and it does not fit in with their dogma, they simply dismiss it. Sometimes they can be so sure that they know the absolute truth that they feel they don't need any more experiences to learn about life. And if that is the case, they can seriously limit themselves and their opportunities for growth. It is wonderful to exhibit self-assurance, self-direction, and single-mindedness. Sagittarius Ascendants can accomplish much that way. However, we never stop learning and growing, and to shut off change will stunt this process.

Your opposite sign, Gemini, is known for being scattered in its thought; it samples a little of this and a little of that, so that it can learn and grow. If you tried opening your mind to let in a few outside thoughts, you might find that there are some worthwhile ideas and concepts floating around, even though they may be different from your own. So maybe your ideas and your moral code will have to be adjusted a bit, but then, you do want to know the truth, don't you? Learn to use the Gemini trait of being open to differing views and opinions and you will come to see change as a good thing, for if in your exploration, you discover some very beneficial truth not already included in your dogma, you will appreciate the fact that you were flexible enough and wise enough to listen.

CAPRICORN ASCENDANT

Capricorn rising people are known for their lack of emotion. They are very detached in their view of the world and in their dealings with others, even those close to them. This ability to be detached can actually work in their favor in the perception of change. They will not dismiss change simply because they didn't order it or because they don't understand it. They will not immediately view it as the enemy or as something to be avoided at all costs. Their view is just the opposite; they will analyze change in a rational, unemotional process. They have an objective perspective. This would indicate that a person with a Capricorn Ascendant should have no trouble perceiving change as positive. And while in some instances this is correct, in many cases it is not.

While you are certainly ambitious, you may not always set your sights in the right direction. Having very lofty goals and reaching them, which is the Capricorn archetype, can relate to either material, earthy goals, or lofty spiritual goals. You can see how the perspective gained from each of these scenarios can be quite different. The perspective of a person entrenched in the material world, wanting, and usually achieving material world objectives, may see a soul-transforming opportunity as being quite unimportant since, from his materialistic perspective, it won't help him in his ascension to the top of the material world. In this way, you may miss out on many transformational possibilities.

Looking to Cancer, the opposite sign of Capricorn, will provide help in this area. Cancer natives are the nurturers of the world and, as such, many times act not only to benefit themselves, but also to benefit those under their care. You would do well to recognize that a change that benefits others as well as yourself can be helpful in your journey to the top of the mountain.

AQUARIUS ASCENDANT

This is the last of the fixed sign Ascendants, and so you probably already recognize the difficulty that these people have in perceiving change as positive. The reason for this is their insistence upon seeing the world in an impersonal fashion. They are known for their universal, all-inclusive view of the world, which is very noble indeed. And yet, they can be very cold and isolated in their relations on a personal level. This would cause them to view change in a very impersonal and cold way, and to walk away from opportunities for change and growth because they can't see these as personal opportunities. Their focus is so universal, that if change is not perceived as benefiting the whole, then it is not worth pursuing.

In order to overcome this universal perception of change, you would do well to study the Leo trait of identifying with the self. Universality and a universal view are, of course, the goals of humanity, but from the perspective of the individual. The individual joins the group, but he is still the individual. And if that individual with the large Leo heart views change through the universal eyes of the Aquarian, change is seen in a more loving, personal way and is perceived as more valuable. You will come to realize that in changing yourself for the better, you are better able to serve humanity, which is your ultimate goal.

PISCES ASCENDANT

Pisces, the last of the mutable signs, would have no problem viewing change as positive in most cases. A person with a Pisces Ascendant feels more than others, because he or she is made up of the components of all the other signs. In fact, a person with a Pisces Ascendant is probably fully aware of the impending changes long before they make their appearance because they are so attuned to what is going on in the universe. A Pisces person flows through life and flows with the changes it constantly presents.

A problem that can arise for you is the perception that, because change is inevitable, you should allow yourself to be swept along with the tide, without exercising any sort of discrimination whatsoever. Part of the problem is that you can so easily feel the pain of others and empathize with those around you, that you sometimes take on more than is required, or become lost in a sea of varying emotional circumstances, some of which are not relevant. So much incoming stimuli can create a condition of clouded vision if you can't separate yourself from everything around you. For this, you need to learn discrimination, one of the key traits of Virgo, your opposite sign. Discrimination will help you to distinguish which changes you need to make for your own personal growth and which changes are unnecessary.

The view from the princess' rock was quite spectacular. The princess, though, had been so engrossed in listening to the little elf that she hadn't paid much attention to her surroundings. But once she lifted her head, and took in the entire landscape, she was amazed at how beautiful it was, and even more amazed that she had not noticed it earlier.

"I am sitting in the most lovely of worlds," she said aloud.

"That you are, my friend," agreed the little elf, and then he pointed out to her some of his favorite sights along the horizon. There was the little lake, an offshoot of the river, where several tiny sailboats were gliding as if on a sheet of ice. There was the flock of white doves flying overhead, and yellow and black butterflies dancing in the foreground. The sky was an indigo blue, with just a few swirls of white clouds. The horizon seemed to go on forever, and it was difficult to ascertain where the land ended and the sky began. When she turned around to see what was behind her, Sebastian pointed out a small range of mountains in the distance.

"You see that purple mountain, the one with the snow-capped peak?"

"How could I miss it?" the princess replied. "It's the tallest and most magnificent."

"It's my home," replied Sebastian.

Of all the most wonderful places to live, mused the princess, the top of a mountain would rank as the most wonderful. Her kingdom, which she had not seen for quite some years now, was a lovely place, but it was not located atop a mountain. She imagined that from Sebastian's mountain, he could look down on the whole world and see everything that was going on at the same time.

"Perspective," replied Sebastian, as if reading her thoughts, "from atop my mountain, I have a very broad view of things."

The princess and Sebastian sat for quite a while in silence, listening to the beautiful sounds, enjoying the fragrant smells and watching life unfold on that lovely summer afternoon. Finally, the princess asked Sebastian if she might someday visit his home.

"It is my greatest wish for you," he told her.

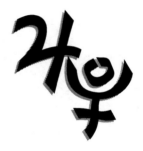

CHAPTER FIVE

JUPITER AND PLUTO IN YOUR CHART: WHAT YOU HAVE TO WORK WITH

Now that we know the basic astrological weight rules, it is time to get to work. We are going to take a look at our natal chart and see what we can learn from it about our weight issues. This chapter will be of particular interest for those people who have always had a weight problem, as opposed to those who were slim as a child and gained weight later in life. People who have always had a weight problem will have indications of it in their natal chart, and by analyzing the natal chart, especially the positions of Jupiter and Pluto, they will be given some very important clues as to what their life is all about, and what they came here to accomplish.

Placement of Jupiter and Pluto in the natal chart by sign relates to the type of enlightenment the individual will encounter in this lifetime or the nature of the item to be relinquished. House placement relates to the area of life where the action will occur. On the following pages, I discuss the significances of natal Jupiter and Pluto in each of the twelve houses and signs. The signs and houses are discussed together because even though signs and houses have different meanings, the effects we feel will be similar. For example, having Jupiter in the second house or having it in the sign of Taurus has very similar manifestations. In both cases, the issue is about values—either what we value or how we value ourselves.

Always remember that, with Jupiter, this enlightenment process adds to or increases your perception. You do not lose what you already have; you just take it to a higher level. You learn to see things in a different, more inclusive way. You view things from a higher perspective. Pluto, on the other hand, asks you to relinquish some person, possession, or point of view, so that you can transform yourself and/or your way of thinking. Where Pluto is concerned, whatever you give up will be replaced with something better—something more in line with your soul's purpose.

Remember, of course, that we are considering both Jupiter and Pluto only as they relate to weight issues, so if you are not having any weight problems, then the following analyses may or may not be applicable to your circumstances.

JUPITER IN ARIES OR THE FIRST HOUSE

This placement of Jupiter enlightens you with a new way of expressing yourself, or a new way of showing initiative. Perhaps you are being asked to look at yourself in a different light. In the past, you might have underestimated yourself or your abilities, and so you are changing your perspective of yourself. Perhaps you don't trust your own intuition, and are being asked by Jupiter to give your intuitive insights the importance they deserve by acting on them. Possibly, there is a pervading problem or issue in your life that can only be solved by taking action. You could be learning to listen to your inner voice and have the courage to follow what it tells you. This position of Jupiter could be asking you to throw away your fear of taking initiative or of acting.

The first house has much to do with how we present ourselves to the world, and so another possible weight-related meaning could be that you are being asked to enlarge your sphere of positive influence on others. It could be that you are being asked to enlarge your leadership role in some way, whether spiritually, emotionally, or mentally. Jupiter in the first or in Aries means that you, as a person, have much to offer and that it is time that you used your tremendous enthusiasm and courage to aid others.

JUPITER IN TAURUS OR THE SECOND HOUSE

Jupiter here may be trying to enlighten you in the area of values. On one level, it may be trying to tell you that you need to value yourself more, and this relates to how you earn a living or what you choose to possess and amass. Jupiter may be asking you to change professions to one that is more in line with what you are really worth and what you have to offer to the world. Jupiter wants you to be paid what you are really worth. This placement could also be related to enlarging your personal or spiritual values, giving you new insights into what is really important to you. You may be asked to look at what you value from a whole new perspective, resulting in a shift in your views of what you want to own and what you want to discard.

If you have had weight issues all of your life and your Jupiter is placed here, think about how you value yourself and what you treasure, because they both need to be lifted to a higher level. Do you feel that you have nothing of value to offer to the world? Look inside yourself, for there is something of value in all of us. We just need to find it and present it to the world, and when we do, we will reap the payment that is appropriate for the value of our offering.

JUPITER IN GEMINI OR THE THIRD HOUSE

Jupiter placed here has much to do with communication, relating to others, learning, and teaching. If you have been plagued with weight problems all your life, Jupiter in this placement may be telling you that you need to learn a new way to communicate and to deal with your surroundings. Or it may be telling you that you need to learn a whole new way of thinking. Adjustments might need to be made in the way you relate to others in your daily environment. Try raising your level of communication or reinventing your thought process. Perhaps your thinking processes just need to be tweaked, or your method of communicating needs to become more inclusive. You might have problems relating to people and you may need to learn to be more inclusive, more open, in your actions.

The gift of Jupiter in the third house is one of a critical mind, and being able to communicate concisely and intelligently with those around you. It's the connection between the higher and lower mind. If you are not using your mind to communicate higher-level thoughts, if you are gossiping too much, or if you are concerned with disseminating the wrong kinds of information, you need to review your communicative processes.

JUPITER IN CANCER OR THE FOURTH HOUSE

Cancer and the fourth house deal with your basic foundation. That foundation can be your home, your early childhood, your family or your basic emotional responses. Constant weight issues for a person with this placement of Jupiter mean that you need to do some work on your basic emotional responses. On a lower level, maybe you need to take a look at your home and raise it to a higher level by inviting others in, or possibly by increasing or enlarging upon its function. Perhaps you need to take the idea of a home or foundation and lift it to a higher level by seeing your home as dwelling inside yourself—as an internal foundation that needs to be strengthened, enlightened, or lifted higher. On another level, you might try looking at your basic emotional responses and see where there are areas for improvement. Or, it could be that your relationship with your family, your mother in particular, needs some work. Also, you should consider defining your relationship with your mother and family in a whole new light, maybe viewing your family from a universal perspective. Perhaps you need to shift your view of family and foundation from personal to universal.

The gift of Jupiter in Cancer or the fourth house is a sensitivity that allows you to relate to those around you and thus to provide nurturance and support to others. If you cannot do this, you have somehow blocked your gift and need to eliminate the negativity that is keeping you from expressing this nurturing and support-ive aspect of yourself.

JUPITER IN LEO OR THE FIFTH HOUSE

The lesson of Jupiter in Leo or the fifth house relates to enlightenment of the self and that which is created by the self. This relates to all creations, be it children, or children of the mind.

Creativity is an expression of our divinity. As above, so below. So when we are displaying creativity, we are showing our godliness, our inner divinity, on a smaller scale. If you are having life-long weight related issues and your natal Jupiter is located in this area of your life, perhaps you need to take a look at your creations. Perhaps you need to lift them to a higher level. Perhaps you are learning to create a broader, more inclusive universe. Maybe you need to change your motives for your creations, giving them a higher purpose. On a lower level, this area of your chart has to do with romance, so you might need to be more inclusive in whom you love. Maybe you need to learn to be more loving. You may need to broaden your perspective not only of whom you love, but also of how your love. Perhaps you need to look at this as going from a personal, self-love to a universal, all-inclusive, spiritual love and go from personal creations, such as children, to creations of the universe, such as books, or art or whatever creation it is that you have within that can benefit the world.

The gift of Jupiter in Leo or the fifth house is the ability to love in a big way, and if you cannot do this, you have blocked that free flow of love. It can be shown most beautifully and joyously through your creations and through those people or things you love.

JUPITER IN VIRGO OR THE SIXTH HOUSE

Consistent weight issues for persons with Jupiter in this area of your chart may have something to do with your daily routine, your daily work, and on a higher level, your service to the world. On a mundane level, the kind of work you do may require that you change to something more appropriate to your basic skills and abilities. On a higher level, the work you do may need to be aligned with your soul's purpose, or your spiritual purpose. Since Jupiter has to do with expansion, it may be that you are in the right area, and that you just need to expand your work a little. You need to take your work to a higher level, make it more inclusive. Your work in the world has a lot to do with your spiritual and moral values, so if what you are doing right now does not relate to your inner moral and spiritual code, you need to fix that. Virgo and the sixth house have much to do with the idea of service, so maybe there needs to be a shift from a self-centered or self-motivated type of service to a more universal concept of service. Also, this area of your chart can relate to health issues, so perhaps that area of your life needs to be addressed. You may need to learn to take better care of yourself or others in your area of concern.

The idea of work and service, of sacrificing oneself to help others, is the essence of this house and sign. You efforts should be focused toward that end in order for the expansiveness represented by Jupiter to be effective.

JUIPTER IN LIBRA OR THE SEVENTH HOUSE

This is the area of personal relationships, namely marriage and business partners. For most of us, the marriage relationship is the one that we are most concerned about, but when analyzing this area, don't forget that it can relate to any close relationship. If you have weight issues and Jupiter is in this area of your natal chart, you need to look at your attitude towards relationships. Do you take your partner for granted? Are you honest and fair in your dealings with your partner? Perhaps you are too controlling in your relationships. This placement of Jupiter is telling you that you need to make a change in how you approach relationships. You need to take your relationships to a higher level, by becoming more detached, more loving toward your mate, or perhaps by looking at the moral or spiritual issues which form the relationship. Maybe you need to redefine the purpose of the relationship, or your idea of what a relationship is.

Another meaning of this placement is that perhaps you are not accepting the benefits that Jupiter has to offer to your relationships. Maybe you are turning your back on opportunities offered by your partner out of fear or indifference, or possibly you aren't aware they exist and need them pointed out to you.

JUPITER IN SCORPIO OR THE EIGHTH HOUSE

If you have been plagued with weight problems all your life and your natal Jupiter is in either Scorpio or the eighth house, you need to take a look at issues relating to death and transformation.

By death, I do not necessarily mean physical death. Jupiter placed here indicates that you have been given many opportunities to "die" in some way and reinvent yourself. The trick, then, is to identify those opportunities and use them correctly. Have you at some point been given the opportunity to change your thinking in a certain area or to change your outlook, especially in areas ruled by the eighth house, such as joint finances, inheritances, insurance issues? Or maybe you have been asked to look at some negative side of yourself and eliminate it once and for all, such as misplaced desires or unnecessary sensitivity, or emotional excess. This can be a very spiritual placement, so possibly it is asking you over the course of your life to increase your spiritual endeavors or your spiritual knowledge. Maybe there is a secret inside of you that needs to come out and be dealt with, and you have been hiding from it. The eighth house relates to money, assets, or anything of value from our partners, so you may be gaining weight because you are missing out on these gifts, and need to be reminded that they exist. Or perhaps, you are taking advantage of your partner's assets or gifts or using them for the wrong purposes. You might not be seeing the value of the partnership, or you may need to align your values with those of your partner.

JUPITER IN SAGITTARIUS OR THE NINTH HOUSE

A natal Jupiter in Sagittarius or the ninth house is especially blessed because Jupiter is the natural ruler of the ninth house, so it functions very well here. The main purpose of this placement is to expand your horizons philosophically, morally and spiritually. Any actions that you take to impede this growth will more than likely result in weight issues. Have you been asked to take a trip to broaden your horizons and refused? Have you passed up the opportunity to expand your consciousness through higher education, seminars, or other educational programs? Have you stopped searching for a philosophical or moral code? Or maybe you have become so set in your beliefs that you refuse to listen to anyone whose ideas are different from your own? Jupiter in this position is giving you the go-ahead to not only expand your own consciousness, but to help others do the same. This is a leadership placement, one in which you are being asked to show others the way to philosophical and spiritual growth. Shunning that responsibility can also create a tremendous "weight." Think about it. Have you been placed in a position where you could help others increase their knowledge, or find their way spiritually? Are you being asked to show others the right way to do things? Is there an issue you need to speak out on but are afraid to do so? Is there an injustice that you need to point out? Jupiter here stands for truth, and you have the ability to live it in a big way. If you are not living your truth, why not?

JUPITER IN CAPRICORN OR THE TENTH HOUSE

Jupiter in Capricorn or the tenth house has a lot to do with your standing in the world. Jupiter here says that you can reach the pinnacle of your career or profession, and it says that you can do it in a big way. Your activities in the world are to always be tempered with kindness and that Jovian spirit of optimism and boundless love. If your natal Jupiter is placed here and you are having weight issues, then you may want to look at how you are presenting yourself to the world through your career or calling. The expansion of consciousness called for here requires that you look inside yourself to find that special gift that only you have and use it for the benefit of all. Not following your true calling can be quite painful, and may be another reason for weight issues. Perhaps you don't know what your true calling is, and again, until you are able to find it, you may have weight issues. The gift of Jupiter in this position is that you have earned the right to rise to the top of the mountain, so to speak, and so if you are not doing what needs to be done to get there, you are not fulfilling your promise. Also, the perspective from the top of the mountain is quite different from down below, and it may be that you need to use this perspective in some new or different way.

JUPITER IN AQUARIUS OR THE ELEVENTH HOUSE

Jupiter in Aquarius or the eleventh house is an indication that you have an innate understanding of the brotherhood of humankind. You are the natural born humanitarian, or are supposed to be. Weight issues for people with this placement may indicate a problem in accepting this premise. Perhaps you have some erroneous ideas or illogical prejudices that need to be rooted out. Maybe you are not as accepting or as tolerant as you should be of the differences in people. Perhaps the issue is just that you are not showing your humanitarian nature in as big a way as you should or could. Working with friends and in group activities should be your strong point. You intuitively know how to combine your energies with those of others to realize a common goal. Are you not as cooperative as you should be? Are you too much of a loner? Are your interests more self-centered than group centered? You may need to enlarge your circle of friends or your group involvements.

This position of Jupiter also allows for the realization of all your hopes and dreams. Weight issues in that area may indicate that adjustments need to be made in what you wish for or dream. Things you may have longed for may no longer be appropriate, or maybe you are selling yourself too short. Perhaps you just need to dream bigger dreams.

JUPITER IN PISCES OR THE TWELFTH HOUSE

This placement indicates compassion for your fellow man and the ability to totally empathize with the experiences of others. Weight issues related to this placement of Jupiter could revolve around either shutting off this compassionate side of yourself, or going to the other extreme and indiscriminately using your gifts. Maybe you are trying to help too many people and need to concentrate your efforts where you can do the most good. Perhaps you are having problems with correctly perceiving reality, and need to make an adjustment. Maybe you have allowed your empathy to turn into self-pity and escapism. This position of Jupiter suggests a lot of psychic and intuitive gifts. Ask yourself if you are using your gifts to the fullest. Could you be using them to aid someone else? Have you turned your back on opportunities to show your intuitive side? Or perhaps you are using your intuitive gifts improperly, maybe for vengeance, or to use or control others? This is a kind and loving placement, and if you are not manifesting that love and kindness in a large way, you will cause a tremendous amount of pain. This placement is asking you to expand your involvement in serving humanity. Use your compassionate nature in ways you have never thought of before.

PLUTO IN ARIES OR THE FIRST HOUSE

Pluto in Aries or the first house is a very powerful position. This placement suggests that you have the strength and willpower to succeed at every task and overcome any foe. In this position, Pluto is asking you to learn to use this power in a positive way, in a way that leads to outcomes for the good of all. Many times, those with weight problems that have this position of Pluto are dealing with issues related to misuse of their personal power. Ask yourself if you are constantly trying to control others, to bend them to your will. If the answer is yes, Pluto here is saying that you must give up those control issues and learn to let go. Rather than trying to make everything go your way, release your desire for control and align your will with that of a higher purpose.

Another problem that can surface with this placement of Pluto relates to emotional excesses. Again, ask yourself if you have become too attached to a particular idea, or person. Perhaps you are determined to win at all costs. Obsessive behavior has to be eliminated. Another possible issue with this placement has to do with how you use your power. Perhaps you have aligned yourself with the wrong idea or the wrong person and so you need to eliminate them so that the correct idea or person can enter your life. Maybe you need to use your powers for something bigger than yourself; in other words, you need to eliminate the smaller, selfish purpose, so that a larger, more inclusive purpose can take its place.

PLUTO IN TAURUS OR THE SECOND HOUSE

Pluto in this position is asking you to eliminate or transform your value system, both the things you value, and how you value yourself. Pluto in this position suggests the ability to earn tremendous amounts of money, and if you are not doing that, it is because you have not discovered what it is that you have of value to offer to the world. What you have to offer to the world is directly related to how you value yourself, so the first thing to do here is throw out your old perception of yourself and begin to build a newer, more correct one. Pluto is forcing you to look deeply inside yourself and bring up all the misconceptions about your personal worth to the forefront and throw them out. Eliminate them completely. Then build a new self, a new sense of self-worth, polish it up, and present it to the world. The kinds of things that you desire are directly related to your personal value, so as you change what you are inside, what you desire will also change. If you desire the wrong kinds of things, you will be forced to give them all up, sometimes rather painfully. If you are hanging onto a lot of weight and you have this position of Pluto, know that you are being asked to give up the things you value for items of greater worth. This position of Pluto may also be asking you to eliminate selfish financial motives or desires, so that you can learn to use your resources for the benefit of all.

PLUTO IN GEMINI OR THE THIRD HOUSE

This placement of Pluto indicates a very focused, perceptive mind and the ability to communicate intelligently, succinctly and with great depth of understanding. Weight issues for a person with this placement may indicate the need to get rid of any faulty thinking or communicative processes. It may indicate that you are not using your mental abilities for the right purposes, and need to eliminate those incorrect purposes so that the appropriate ones can surface. For instance, ask yourself if you are using your astute mental powers to hurt others, possibly through scheming, plotting, etc. Wrong use of Plutonian energy many times relates to control and, in this case, control of others with your mental prowess. Are you using your communication skills to dominate or control others, or to sway them to your way of thinking? Are you overly aggressive in pushing your opinions on others? Are you obsessed with your opinions and ideas? All of these types of behavior need to be eliminated, and replaced with more appropriate uses for your tremendous powers of thought.

PLUTO IN CANCER OR THE FOURTH HOUSE

Pluto in Cancer or the fourth house is an indication of someone who is very well connected with his or her emotional and psychological base or foundation. Weight issues for someone with this placement of Pluto may relate to the fact that you are so connected with your inner emotions that you are obsessed with them and with your most basic desires. Obsessions of any kind need to be eliminated, and transformed into more appropriate behavior. Obsessions with emotional desires can be changed into compassionate and nurturing behavior simply by transforming the focus of the obsession from one of control and inflexibility to one of healing and peace. If you suffer from an inordinate amount of feelings of jealousy, selfishness and possessiveness, or other negative emotions, you are being asked to release these emotions and replace them with love and compassion. Intense emotions can be used for good or ill. Ask yourself how you are using yours. If you don't like the answer you receive, work on eliminating the inappropriate uses and find good ones.

PLUTO IN LEO OR THE FIFTH HOUSE

Children, creativity, and intense heartfelt love come with this placement of Pluto. One can be so intensely involved with one's children or creative ideas, that obsession can set in. If that is the case, a lifelong battle with weight could result from refusing to overcome these obsessions. It is one thing to love and care for a child, whether a real child or a child of the mind. But if you find yourself trying to control the movements and thoughts of your child, or if you find that you are so obsessed with your creation that you cannot bear to let it loose in the world, then you have gone overboard. Pluto in this position will require that you relinquish the obsessive control you have, so that your creations can reach their full potential. When you try to keep them all to yourself, you are impeding their growth, either the growth of your child or the growth of your ideas. Let them go and your beautiful creations can be shared with the world. Eliminate your jealousy and possessiveness from your being. Many times people ask, "What is the 'something better' that I will receive when I let go of whatever it is that Pluto is asking of me?" The answer, in this case, is that you will receive more love because you have shared something beautiful with an appreciative world. This position of Pluto shows you have the potential to warm and heal others through your creative abilities, so if you are not using your powers to do that, you will be required to eliminate the cause of the blockage.

PLUTO IN VIRGO OR THE SIXTH HOUSE

Intensity is always an appropriate word for Pluto and, in this case, the intensity can be applied to your devotion to your work and service to others. This position implies great healing powers due to the relation of Virgo and the sixth house to health issues, and critical thinking powers as well, due to the connection with Mercury. The kind of work that you do and how you serve your community is quite important here. If you are having weight issues and your Pluto is placed here, you might want to take a look at your daily routine. Are you in the correct line of work? Are you running from opportunities to use your abilities to help or serve others? Or maybe there are health issues involved. How is your personal hygiene? Do you take care of yourself the way you should? You have much resourcefulness and willpower that can work wonders in these areas. How are you using that willpower? Are you using it to hurt others? Are you overly discriminating against people you find offensive rather than serving all? Are you separating yourself from those you feel are not quite up to your standards? Any of these negative tendencies must be eliminated, and a new, more inclusive attitude towards service must take its place.

PLUTO IN LIBRA OR THE SEVENTH HOUSE

Pluto in this position bestows intensity in the area of partnerships and close personal relationships. Pluto's transformative powers work in this area of your chart to eliminate any unhealthy relationship issues. The obvious ones are being overly controlling or possessive, and of course, if you are in a relationship where you are either the controller or the controllee, prepare to have the relationship totally overhauled, maybe even eliminated. But relationships develop in many ways, and people relate to each other for a variety of reasons. Some of the reasons we come together are very good—for instance, common goals, shared interests, etc. But some of the reasons we come together have to do with very sinister motives, such as ambition, greed, coercion, etc. Sometimes we are unaware of the motivating forces behind our relationships, and Pluto brings these underlying issues to the surface so that we can face them and eliminate them. If you have been struggling with weight issues for a long time and your Pluto is placed here, ask yourself if you have been trying to hold onto a deteriorating relationship, one you should have exited from many years ago. Perhaps you are taking your mate for granted, or are exhibiting other traits which do not put you in the best light as a partner. Maybe honesty in relationships is an issue for you and needs to be addressed. Another possibility is that you just need to allow Pluto to take you to the depths so that he can show you what you truly need in a mate because you are unsure at this time or have been making wrong choices. Whatever the transformation, once you make it, expect your relationships to be one hundred percent improved.

PLUTO IN SCORPIO OR THE EIGHTH HOUSE

Pluto can be quite powerful in this placement for the eighth house is Pluto's natural home. Expect a life of constant change and transformation in areas related to deep-seated neuroses or life-threatening negative behaviors. A positive side to this placement is that it is indicative of an individual with intense personal power, comparable to those with Pluto in the first house or Aries. Problems with weight, then, would relate to misuse of this power, or attempts to thwart any of the numerous life transformations this placement brings. They can cover a variety of areas in your life, so it may be difficult to pin down exactly where Pluto is requiring you to do the work. You can help narrow the field by looking at the things, people, beliefs, and feelings you are most attached to, for these are the things you will most likely end up giving up. Possible issues could be finances, which seem to often be in a state of fluctuation for those with this placement. You might want to ask yourself why that is so. Maybe your attitude toward money, especially joint finances and unearned income, needs to be revamped. Perhaps yours is a life of constantly striving to find the answers to the deeper mysteries of life, such as birth and death, and the transformation may be one of eliminating outdated personal values and priorities for more timeless and spiritually inclined ones.

PLUTO IN SAGITTARIUS OR THE NINTH HOUSE

Pluto in Sagittarius or the ninth house indicates a life of intense spiritual expansion. There is a deep and profound search for basic truths, and a desire to develop a life philosophy or moral code. People with this placement will, therefore, constantly shift their view of the world, and broaden their knowledge and wisdom. Weight issues related to this placement of Pluto would have to do with either fighting the enlightening experiences, or becoming so obsessed with one's own beliefs as to try to force them on others. With regards to the first issue, that of fighting your spiritual progress, you should be able to tell if you are guilty of this. Have you had opportunities to expand your knowledge through travel, or some educational pursuit, and refused to even consider them? Sometimes, this is because you are stuck in a particular belief system, one that needs to be either completely updated or eliminated altogether. Again, if you are obsessed with your religious, spiritual or moral beliefs, then more than likely, they are the target of Pluto. All obsessions have to be eliminated, so that a healthier attitude can take its place. This placement of Pluto also relates to publishing and legal issues, so you may find yourself being asked to make major adjustments or transformations in these areas of your life.

PLUTO IN CAPRICORN OR THE TENTH HOUSE

Pluto in Capricorn or the tenth house means major transformations throughout your life in your career or profession, and your status in the outside world. Who people think you are will change drastically as your life proceeds, and you will find that who you think you are today won't make sense ten years from now. This is a natural and desirable transformation, and so anything you do to fight it will only create problems. If you are fighting weight and your Pluto is in this area of your chart, look to see if you are presenting yourself to the world in a way that is most in line with who you are and with your particular talents. This placement of Pluto will make you look deep inside yourself to find your true life's mission—that particular contribution to the world that only you can make. Finding it for some is quite easy; for others it takes a long, long time. Until you find it, your career will be constantly changing, in a sometimes frustrating and often painful process. If you fight to stay in a career because it is comfortable, it will most likely be yanked away from you in true Plutonian fashion. Another effect of fighting Pluto's wishes for you is to find yourself involved in public scandals or in situations where you are publicly humiliated or disgraced. Weight issues involving Pluto in the tenth can only be resolved if one is willing to look deep inside, find their true calling, and use their immense Plutonian energy to fulfill it.

PLUTO IN AQUARIUS OR THE ELEVENTH HOUSE

Pluto in Aquarius or the eleventh house indicates a deep commitment to friendships and group involvement. The kinds of friends we choose and the groups we belong to have a lot to do with our hopes and wishes. We want friends and associates who will support us in our endeavors and who have similar views and goals. When a friendship or group has outlived its usefulness in our life, we need to move on, for if we stay in relationships that no longer serve a purpose, we are stunting our own growth. Persons with this placement of Pluto who are dealing with weight issues need to take a look at the people and organizations in their lives and assess whether or not they are appropriate for where they are currently in their evolutionary cycle. Ask yourself if there are people in your life who are holding you back, or if you belong to organizations whose goals you no longer support. Allow Pluto to take you to the depths of your soul so that you can determine what you truly want from life. Once you know what your innermost hopes and wishes are, Pluto shows you how to pursue them with a vengeance. Obviously, if you are fighting this process, or if you know what your true hopes and dreams are and are not pursuing them, you will be fighting this transformational process and will pay in many ways. Let go of people or organizations not in line with your current goals. Release old, worn out dreams and replace them with more appropriate ones.

PLUTO IN PISCES OR THE TWELFTH HOUSE

Pluto in Pisces or in the twelfth house promises a life full of intense psychological examination, and a constant process of eliminating subconscious memories, fears and phobias. With this placement of Pisces, we continually confront our deepest nature, with the purpose of transforming our buried secrets into hidden treasures. This is a powerfully introspective placement, and allows the native to penetrate his inner self. This placement is asking you to eliminate everything in your subconscious that is holding you back from the true expression of your soul. Release these inner fears and stop dragging them around with you. True soul expression for the person with this placement involves the compassionate serving of humanity. This is the placement of the true healer, for there is much power here to help others. If you have this placement and are not able to focus your Pluto intensity on helping others, you must determine what psychological issues are holding you back and eliminate them. If not eliminated, these issues may manifest as weight problems.

The next information you want to glean from your natal chart has to do with the relationship of Jupiter and Pluto to the other planets. By studying the aspects that these two planets make to the other planets in your natal chart, and to each other, you can determine what kind of energy you have to work with in overcoming your weight issues. Perhaps you have more power than you thought, or perhaps you are just using the energy in the wrong way. Soft aspects refer to the trine, sextile and conjunction. Hard aspects are the square, opposition and inconjunct (quincunx). Again, we are looking at these energy combinations strictly in terms of how they relate to weight control and weight issues.

JUPITER AND THE SUN

This can be a very difficult combination where weight is concerned. The purpose of this aspect is to allow an expansion, or growth in consciousness, of the personality. This is because, on the personality level, Jupiter and the Sun combine to signify a sense of tremendous optimism and a broadness of spirit. Used improperly, though, this energy combination can lead to a tendency towards excesses where personal expression is concerned. Hard aspects are more difficult, (almost always resulting in problems with excesses and over indulgence) but sometimes even the soft aspects can indicate weight issues. An over-inflated personality, thinking too highly of oneself, and self-centeredness can all result from improper use of these energies. The reins need to be pulled in a little and the energies should be focused away from the personal self and towards development of one's inner or soul purpose. An over-inflated ego almost always results in an overweight physical body.

JUPITER AND THE MOON

This is another very difficult combination in terms of weight control. This time, the excesses go much deeper than the personality level. They go down to the very emotional and psychological foundation, and are much harder to rein in and control, especially in the case of hard aspects. An excess of emotions can manifest as an excess of weight if the emotional body has been inflated or enlarged. These energies together, if inappropriately directed, can cause one to become an emotional wreck. The beauty of this combination is that it can allow an expansion of one's intuitional nature, but only after the negative emotional excesses have been subdued. This positive intuitional expansion is usually possible with the trine and sextile, and is quite pronounced with the conjunction. If you have this in hard aspect, the energies must be lifted to a higher plane, so that they can be used as they were intended, not to over emphasize negative emotions, but to beautifully expand your ability to innately understand the universe and your place in it.

JUPITER AND MERCURY

This combination indicates an expansive intellect, and outstanding communication skills. The energy combination can, if used correctly, lead to new intellectual concepts and insights that the native can easily share with others. Mercury, as messenger of the gods, teaches us how to connect with our higher intellect and beyond. We can see the vision of our higher self, our goals, our life's purpose, and we can then transmit this information to others using Jupiter's power to relate to others in a large way. This energy combination implies clear, concise thought, for you can see clearly where you are going and express it in a way that others can understand. You can easily relate one thing to another, and one person to another, thanks to Jupiter's optimism and generosity and Mercury's insight. Negative use of this energy, which can occur with hard aspects, results in a skewed vision, and the resultant incorrect dissemination of ideas and thoughts. It can also produce a person who gossips or talks too much, or someone who communicates inaccuracies. To alleviate the problems that can arise with the hard aspects, try to remember, before you open your mouth or put pen to paper, to take the higher road because you want to communicate the higher vision.

JUPITER AND VENUS

Jupiter and Venus can be another challenging combination where weight is concerned because of Venus's magnetism and tendency toward indulging one's desires and Jupiter's powers of expansion. If we attract the wrong things to ourselves, and we do it in a big way, which Jupiter implies, we can be saddled with a lot of extra, unwanted baggage. The positive power represented by these two planets creates a tremendous opportunity to express love to our fellow humans in a magnanimous way. Another way of saying this, is that with this combination, we are literally overflowing with love. So the question is what is it that we love? In the case of the hard aspects, this combination can mean that we have a tremendous love for ourselves, or for our desires, and that we need to channel that energy into a higher type of love or desire. Love of self can be transformed into love of others, and desire can be transformed into aspiration.

JUPITER AND MARS

This combination normally does not signify weight issues, but it can represent a powerful force if you are dealing with weight problems indicated by other aspects and placements of Jupiter and Pluto. Jupiter and Mars motifs combine to give you an almost warrior-like exuberance. You give yourself wholeheartedly to your cause and are unwavering in your commitment. Indeed, you are willing to fight to the death for what you believe is right and just. You can see how, if properly placed, this combination suggests that you can make great strides in reaching your goals. You feel you can conquer anything, defeat any foe. Obviously, you can see how a problem can arise with hard aspects, for you may be wasting this energy if you are fighting for the wrong causes. This combination works best when you are using it to achieve moral or spiritual growth.

JUPITER AND SATURN

Combining the planet of expansion and the planet of restriction results in a sort of standoff. The optimism of Jupiter is tempered by the seriousness of Saturn, and so one walks the middle road. This combination is unique in that both the soft and hard aspects have pretty much the same significance. Saturn is related to karma and therefore is key to many of the difficult or seemingly strange circumstances and relationships that develop in our lives, the purpose being to overcome past negative karma by making more appropriate choices this time around. The energies of Jupiter and Saturn can be used optimistically and responsibly, to face the challenging opportunities and situations that have been created for our spiritual growth.

JUPITER AND URANUS

Jupiter encourages us to broaden our horizons, and Uranus emphasizes our drive for individuality and our need to explore alternatives, so the combination works very well together, especially in the soft aspects. With conjunctions, trines and sextiles of these two planets, the individual may be totally aware of everything that is unexplored and just waiting to be discovered. There is a limitless thirst for new and unique experiences. Accompanying feelings of freedom and uniqueness pervade the individual and there is an excitement that comes from simply being alive. This planetary combination is wonderful for the promotion of spiritual growth, because the native is not afraid of change. However, this combination is not always used that way in the case of the hard aspects. Sometimes it is indicative of individuals who choose to be different just for the sake of being different—for shock value, or just plain rebelliousness. In those cases, the individual needs to take a look at what he is really trying to accomplish with his life and determine if his actions are supportive.

JUPITER AND NEPTUNE

Neptune, representing our highest ideals, and Jupiter, representing soul growth and expansion, can combine to represent an enormous desire to do good and compassionate work in the world. Or, this combination can signify just the opposite. With the hard aspects, the individual may seek escape from his higher purpose through all sorts of negative influences, such as drug or alcohol abuse, or self-delusion. We may hide out from our obligation to the world by living in our own dream world, self-imposed isolation, or obsession with our subconscious nature to the point that we have a hard time coming back down to earth. This escapism, although difficult, can be overcome by doing what comes naturally to those with the soft aspects of this planetary combination, namely, by being enormously loving and generous to those with whom we come into contact and by staying connected with our soul purpose.

JUPITER AND PLUTO

When the motifs of the largest and smallest planet combine, you have an intense amount of power with enormous depth and breadth. This combination is quite similar to that of the combination of Mars and Jupiter, except that it is more intense. "Death to the enemy" would accurately describe the sentiments of one with this energy combination, as the person would exert all of his efforts to eliminate any undesirable trait or person or situation from his life that stood in his way. This can be a very positive combination where soul growth is concerned, for the enormous intensity present here pretty much guarantees that all hindrances to soul growth and consciousness raising will be rooted out and eliminated. However, used incorrectly, this combination can create havoc, for in hard aspects, it may end up destroying something of value. It is extremely important that this energy be focused on the right target.

PLUTO AND THE SUN

This combination indicates enormous willpower, resourcefulness and personal power. The person who has these planets in aspect, whether hard or soft, is able to easily achieve his goals and desires, because he can intently focus on making them happen. Full self-expression is never a problem, for the native can always find a way to overcome any obstacles in his path. With the soft aspects, the native has no qualms about eliminating unwanted or undesirable traits, people or situations from his life, for he innately understands why they have to go. With hard aspects, though, he may use his great resourcefulness and personal power to find clever and ingenious ways to avoid what he perceives as unwanted change or growth. Incorrect use of this planetary combination can be indicative of an individual who is controlling, obsessive and unyielding in his positions. Since the Sun is involved here, there can be weight issues involved with this combination in hard aspects if the individual holds onto that which should be released.

PLUTO AND THE MOON

This planetary combination represents energies that are psychic and probing, giving the native an intensely introspective nature. Soft aspects imply that the person can delve into the depths of his emotional and psychological nature and completely rid himself of negative feelings and emotions. Total control of the emotional nature is possible, so that the individual is then free to listen to his intuition, and follow its guidance. The hard aspects signify intensified emotions. It may be harder to eliminate them, for the individual becomes obsessed with his feelings, and is so strongly attached to them that he will fight to retain them. The hard aspects can, therefore, contribute to weight gain, for emotional intensity can show up in the physical realm as weight.

PLUTO AND MERCURY

This combination symbolizes a very shrewd mind, and the individual can either use his abilities for good or ill. Normally, aspects between these two planets do not relate to weight issues, although it is conceivable that if one were to hold on to outdated or incorrect patterns of thinking, communicating, or relating to others, that it could manifest as excess weight. The same may occur if wrong uses are made of one's mental and communicative capacities. The best use of this aspect is to blend your acute perceptions and vast knowledge in order to become balanced in your thinking and to be able to recognize truth. This combination of energies gives you tremendous depth of vision, and the ability to communicate that vision to others.

PLUTO AND VENUS

This combination marries Pluto's intensity with Venus' love nature. As related to weight, this combination, used negatively, causes one to be passionately devoted to his emotions and his desires, and thus, can cause the manifestation of excess weight. The soft aspects imply that one can exhibit the higher level of desires and the love nature, while hard aspects often showcase deep, intense, baser desires. The symbolic transformative quality of Pluto allows for the elimination of these powerful and intense feelings, but only if the individual is willing. If the individual uses the energies represented by this planetary combination correctly, he can develop a very healthy attitude towards love and other passions, and he will know how to show love to others.

PLUTO AND MARS

Individuals with these two planets in hard aspect in their charts should know that this could be a very dangerous combination if used incorrectly. The aggressive and violent qualities of Mars combined with the intensity and obsession of Pluto can create a scenario where violence, illegal acts, or cruelty show themselves. This, of course, would be the extreme, but is quite possible, for this is a combination of powerful desires and strong will. Used correctly, this combination signifies a person with potent energy to accomplish anything, and can be a great aid in releasing any negative emotions or thoughts caused by other weight related aspects.

PLUTO AND JUPITER
See JUPITER AND PLUTO above.

PLUTO AND SATURN
Intensity and discipline combine to produce maturity, responsibility and resourcefulness. When carried overboard, as can happen with the hard aspects, this person can have an overly developed sense of duty, or can feel that life is extremely hard and difficult. This is due to the fact that Saturn, especially with hard aspects, relates to karmic debt. This energy, though, can be used positively whether in hard or soft aspects, if the individual chooses to use the traits of extreme discipline and responsibility to work on eliminating negative aspects of the self that are causing weight issues.

PLUTO AND URANUS
This is a most dynamic combination of intensity and electricity. The result can be a dazzling display of personal power. Uranus represents changes, and Pluto implies that these changes will be life transforming. The result is an individual who feels intensely independent and free, and is totally open to change for the sake of personal and soul growth. Normally this combination would not be associated with any major weight issues, but the hard aspects would be more likely to indicate problems revolving around improper use of these energies, i.e., an overly rebellious nature, or being different just to be different or to get attention. This aspect can be used positively to innovate new ideas and behaviors, and so can aid in eliminating negative thoughts, ideas and behavior patterns.

PLUTO AND NEPTUNE

Pluto in aspect with Neptune is a powerfully spiritual combination. It resonates the transformative powers of the soul in order to manifest the highest, idealized version of itself. Weight control can be an issue, though, because Neptune can symbolize clouded perceptions and confusion regarding the idealized version of the self. Positive aspects suggest the person can penetrate the depths of his soul and discover his true self; hard aspects may correlate with being kept in the dark. With Neptune, there is always a choice of reaching for the higher or lower self. If the latter is chosen, one hides from oneself in a cloud of foggy thinking, or remains constantly in alcohol- or drug-induced states so as not to face reality. Positive use of the energy, that is, to find one's true spiritual nature and use it for the benefit of all, will eliminate any negative weight issues.

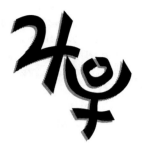

CHAPTER SIX

TRANSITS OF JUPITER AND PLUTO TELL US WHAT THEY WANT

Now it is time to look at the causes of recent weight gain. Suppose you had never had any weight problems until you were in your thirties. Before that time, you may have had a few minor weight fluctuations, but nothing you couldn't handle. Then something happened a few years ago (and you can probably pinpoint the time when the problems began) that caused you to gain a lot of weight and you have never been able to get rid of it. If you identify with this situation, then this chapter is for you because we are going to look at weight from the perspective of timing.

NOT FOR WOMEN ONLY

Now, understand that I am not talking about the infamous weight that a lot of women gain during pregnancy. I am referring to that weight that you just can't seem to lose no matter what you do, even though your child is already ten years old. If it has been years and you have not been able to lose the weight from the birth of a child, there is definitely a deeper cause. More than likely, there was a transit going on around the time of the pregnancy that will explain the tenaciousness of the extra poundage, and hopefully, you can discover it here.

Related to this type of weight gain is the extra weight some women deal with when going through menopause. This situation is similar to that of pregnancy; while the tendency is definitely there to gain weight during this time of your life, there is usually a specific, underlying reason for the weight gain, and you have to search for it just as in any other situation. Think about it. Some women go through menopause without any hot flashes or weight gain, or any other problems and there is a reason why. The rules we have been discussing all along relate to menopause as well.

Finally, I want to point out another phenomena related to weight and giving birth, the creative kind. It has been my experience, and the experience of several of my friends who do something creative such as writing or painting for a living, that during the creation process, there could be a tendency to put on weight. It is as if the extra poundage relates to the creative "child" within and, until it is finally born, we carry that unexpressed creativity as excess poundage. This is not contrary to what I stated above about pregnancy. This phenomenon actually confirms it. The child within does weigh something and until it is born, it is extra weight that we as the mother carry. Once it is born, though, and this has always been my experience with writing, the birth of the artistic or creative endeavor allows for a tremendous loss of weight—mentally, emotionally, spiritually, and physically. If we continue to carry extra weight long after the creative process has been completed, then, just as with a pregnancy, we must look to other causes for the excess weight. To do that requires that we study the transits of Jupiter and Pluto.

WHAT IS A TRANSIT?

First of all, I need to explain just exactly what astrologers mean when they speak of transits. The natal chart shows the placement of the planets at the exact moment you were born, but the planets are constantly moving in their own distinct orbits at their own differing speeds. A transit describes the current movement of the planets as they pass through the signs and houses of your astrological chart.

Some planets move more quickly than others, so they can pass through the houses and signs of your chart many, many times during your life. These faster moving planets are called the personal planets, since their significance is more personal in

nature and comes and goes quickly because of the rapid movement of the planets involved. The personal planets, or inner
planets, are the Sun, Moon, Mercury, Venus, and Mars. The outer
planets, starting with Jupiter, have longer orbits, and thus, spend
a longer time in each of the houses and signs in your chart. Therefore, their significance is greater. For example, Jupiter spends a
year in each sign, and Pluto can spend from 12 to 31 years in any
one sign. That is a long enough time to truly transform even the
toughest individuals.

The second thing to remember about transits is that they
represent specific issues and drives that you are dealing with for a
limited period of time—the length of time of the transit. It is as if
a flashlight is illuminating a particular area of your life for a
specific reason and period of time. We are to make the most of
this by first understanding the purpose of the lighted period, and
then what we are supposed to do within this limited time frame.
Hopefully, the descriptions of the implications of Jupiter and Pluto
through the signs and houses in Chapter Five have given you
insight as to the purpose of the transit. The only thing left for you
to figure out is how to put the energies, symbolized by these two
planets, to good use in the time frame provided.

ASPECTS TO TRANSITING PLANETS

As Pluto and Jupiter are traveling through your chart, they
may be connecting with your natal planets by aspect. Whenever
this happens, their significance in the particular house or sign they
are in becomes even stronger, and this significance or influence is
colored by the qualities of the planet they are aspecting. For
instance, if Pluto has been transiting your sixth house of work and
service for the last three years, you may have noticed that you
have become more interested in your health, and have begun
taking better care of yourself. But if, in its journey through your
sixth house, Pluto squares your natal Moon, suddenly health
issues really jump to the forefront, as you are being asked to deal
with a health issue that perhaps you were not even aware of
before. Pluto indicates issues being brought to the surface so that
you can deal with them, and the Moon indicates sensitivity to aid

in bringing these same deeply buried psychological issues to the forefront. Whenever the Moon is involved, issues fundamental to your emotional nature are implied, and depending on the types of issues, facing them may be very painful. The fact that the aspect is a square would indicate that this could indeed be a very difficult time in one's life, and if the individual chose the indirect route of escapism instead of facing the issues head on, very painful or very "heavy" results could manifest. An aspect like this could add a lot of pounds to the process unless the individual going through the process chooses to face it head on rather than remaining passive and clinging to outdated relationships and situations.

Transits of Jupiter can indicate the same kind of "heavy" results if the native chooses the escapism route. However, with Jupiter, the implied significance of the transit won't be as painful. It will seem to the person that his life is becoming one of extremes. Issues related to the area of his life being transited by Jupiter may seem a little out of control. If Jupiter were squaring the Moon, for example, rather than bringing to the surface uncomfortable, sub-conscious issues, the Moon and Jupiter could indicate an excess of these uncomfortable emotional or psychological issues so that, at some point, the individual might feel as if he were a walking emotional time bomb, ready to explode at any moment.

The beauty of transits, though, is that they do eventually end. And so, the feeling of being tightly wound emotionally as indicated by Jupiter squaring the Moon, or of having to deal with psychological issues that Pluto dredges up, does eventually pass. How well you did in handling the situation will be indicated physically by how you look after the transit is over. Of course, you know by now that if you didn't handle the situation well, you could be left with a souvenir of excess weight to remind you of what you failed to do when asked.

OTHER PLANETARY HELPERS

Is it too late to fix things once the transit has passed? Absolutely not. As a matter of fact, it is sometimes easier to do the work later on in your life when you have better transits and aspects. What I mean is that certain other planets represent qualities that are more in line with making changes and making progress than are those indicated by Jupiter and Pluto. Saturn transits, for instance, are wonderful for times when you need to be disciplined. So, if you missed out on the opportunity to lose weight under a Pluto transit because you just couldn't bring yourself to give up whatever it was that Pluto was asking you to rid yourself of, look to your next Saturn transit to attempt to tackle the problem and you will discover that if you have the right intention, you can accomplish much. Saturn represents the task-master, and if you are willing to "bite the bullet" and do the hard work, then success is pretty much assured.

Another planet that symbolizes energies that can help you succeed where you failed under Jupiter and Pluto is the mysterious planet Neptune. Neptune transits are wonderful for helping you to understand meanings or to make things clear. I can see you scratching your head. Traditional astrology says that Neptune makes things less clear and that it can cloud your judgment and, in certain circumstances, this is correct. But Neptune is the planet of inspiration and can indicate divine insight and intuition if you know how to ask for it. Neptune allows you to see the best and the worst in yourself. By looking for the very best that you can be, Neptunian motifs can many times show you what needs to be done in order to get there. On the other hand, by looking towards your lowest self, the drives represented by Neptune can help take you there also.

For example, Neptune transiting your seventh house indicates what you want in an ideal partner, or shows you how you can be one. If, however, you chose to resist the urge to reach for the heights, and seek escapism instead, Neptune can be indicative of delusional thinking, causing you to believe that someone is an ideal partner when in fact he or she is the very worst possible partner for you. Neptune transits can also indicate that you have deluded yourself into thinking that your behavior in a relationship is quite appropriate when it fact it is not. If you have been having problems with your weight and Neptune is going to be making a major aspect to either Jupiter or Pluto, or it is transiting the same house as either transiting or natal Jupiter or Pluto, pay particular attention to your dreams, your intuitive feelings and your hunches. They may have a tremendous bearing on the situation and may help you remedy it.

The third outer planet that can sometimes benefit you once you have passed a Jupiter or Pluto transit is the mighty Uranus. Uranus represents sudden, unexpected and often disruptive energy. That is, whenever you know that Uranus is going to be active in your chart, expect the unexpected. And expect it to make its presence known loudly and clearly. Uranus in connection with Jupiter indicates things happening very quickly, and working with Pluto, it can indicate a forcing of the issue involved which often results in the item surfacing faster than it would have under Pluto's influence alone. Suppose, for example, that transiting Pluto has recently visited your eighth house; perhaps you added some extra weight as a result, and Uranus is following Pluto. Since Uranus will cover the same ground, expect the issue to become even more prominent than before. Uranus transiting this already heavily trodden area of your life indicates that you will probably find it very difficult to hold onto any outdated ideas or relationships that you may have chosen to hold onto during the Pluto transit. Uranus entering the scene adds a sense of urgency or perhaps a series of events that you may feel are not under your control, to assist you in completing the unfinished business from the Pluto aspect. However, if Uranus had preceded Pluto in aspecting that particular area of your chart, it would have been indicative of disruption in that area of your life; by the time Pluto arrived, you would probably have already done much of the work.

The bottom line is, if you wanted to make a change using the energies representative of a Pluto or Jupiter transit and just didn't have the courage to do it at the time, never fear, for the energies symbolized by Uranus will allow you to finish the task if you so choose. However, keep in mind that you may want to do the job yourself, without Uranus's help, because at least you will feel that you have more control over the way in which things happen. If you wait for Uranus to do it, things may be a bit more disruptive. Uranus is indicative of feeling as if circumstances are out of your control and that you are merely watching the demolition from the sidelines.

SIMILARITIES BETWEEN NATAL AND TRANSITING JUPITER AND PLUTO

Hopefully, you can see how Saturn, Neptune and Uranus can all be very helpful in working through your Pluto or Jupiter issues if they visit the same area of your chart. What do you do, though, if you aren't going to have any help from these three planets in the near future? Are you just stuck with that extra poundage until the next time Jupiter or Pluto shows up in that area? Thankfully, the answer again is no. You need to approach the problem of the excess weight as if it were given to you by your natal chart, and use the tools given to you in Chapter Five.

Once you have gone through a Jupiter or Pluto transit and have manifested the extra weight signifying the internalization of an issue that should have been eliminated or enlightened in some way, you are really in the same place as if you had been born with that tendency. The only recourse is to try to figure out what it was that they wanted you to do, and then do it. Without help from Saturn, Neptune and Uranus, it will be harder, but that is the result of the choice you made. The easiest time to make the change was during the original Jupiter or Pluto transit. Everything was set up perfectly to make the change but you fought it, so now you will have to work a little harder to succeed.

But you can succeed. Let me give you some examples. Suppose you have been separated from your family. Suppose the separation was caused by a major argument you had ten years ago at Christmas and you have refused to have any contact with them since. This split has been eating at you for many years and deep down inside you know that you want to work things out but your pride will not allow you to do so. Jupiter recently transited your fourth house of home and family, trying to get you to rise above the pettiness that caused the split with your family, and to look at the situation from a different perspective. During the transit, your sister sent you a card saying that everyone in the family misses you and wants to talk to you to work out the differences, which you still feel are irreconcilable. And not only that, your feelings are still hurt after all these years, and you just cannot forgive them. Your sister presented you with an opportunity during the Jupiter transit to redress this issue but you fought this idea, and instead chose to continue to harbor your anger and unforgiving attitude. You constantly fed this anger by eating and eating the entire year of the transit. As a result, you now weigh fifteen pounds more than you did a year ago, and you are still not speaking to anyone in your immediate family. The easy opportunity has passed, so you will have to create your own opportunities if you are to remedy this situation. However you have to do it, you will have to be the one who initiates some sort of reconciliatory meeting, and you will have to do it without the aid of beneficial Jupiterian energies. You can do it but it will be harder.

Transiting Jupiter and Pluto have basically the same meaning in the signs and houses as natal Jupiter and Pluto, and since we looked at them in Chapter Five, I will not go through them again here. There is a major difference though—with transits there is more of a sense of urgency. The idea of a limited amount of time is the overriding issue wherever transits are involved. With a natal chart placement, you have the luxury of being able to work on certain issues your entire life, but with transits (as well as progressions which you will learn about in the next chapter) you don't have the opportunity to work on certain issues until you reach a particular age or point in your development. In interpreting a transit, a critical question you need to ask yourself is why this particular event is happening to you at this particular time in your life. Being able to answer that question can sometimes help you in understanding the nature and purpose of the change and make it easier for you to assimilate it.

WHEN TRANSITING JUPITER AND PLUTO ASPECT NATAL JUPITER AND PLUTO

One way of looking at the distinction between the natal placement of Jupiter and Pluto and transits of these same planets is that the natal placement represents issues that you have been struggling with for many lifetimes, and that transits are issues that are not really ingrained in your personality yet and can be remedied if the proper work is done during the transit. But what does it mean if transiting Jupiter and Pluto are affecting the same areas as your natal Jupiter and Pluto?

If you gain weight during a transit of Jupiter and it is going through the house of its natal placement, this is then a very important transit, and affords you the opportunity to really fix this problem once and for all. Pluto, because it travels so much more slowly than Jupiter, will not transit the house of its natal placement during your lifetime, but it will make aspects to your natal Pluto, and again, these aspects are opportunities to make tremendous strides in those areas. If your natal Pluto is in your fifth house, for instance, and transiting Pluto will be squaring it this year, pay close attention to the issues that present themselves at that time; resolve them correctly and you should be able to eliminate your weight issue for good.

The most important thing to remember about transits is that once they are over, they are over. Whatever it is that they were trying to teach you ends when the transit ends. So do not waste them. This is why the study of astrology is so important. Astrology gives you the ability to identify major transits before they happen so that you can prepare for them. While I am not saying that you only have one chance to make a major change in your life, I am saying that you should not waste opportunities, for you may have to wait a long time for the next one to arrive. In some cases, opportunities don't arrive again, especially in the case of Pluto. So, realize that transits of Jupiter and Pluto are major blessings; they are opportunities for soul growth as well as physical, mental and emotional growth.

JUPITER AND PLUTO IN THE LAST DEGREES

Another important issue regarding transits relates to the position of the transiting planet. If Jupiter or Pluto is transiting the last degree of a sign, that is, the 29th degree, or the last degree of a house (this differs from chart to chart) then the influence of the planet is extremely powerful and thus this is the best time for achieving results. Right before a planet leaves a sign or a house, it is as if the planet shoots out one last major thrust of energy, so that if you haven't made the suggested change, you can still do so in a big way. This last thrust of energy can either spell major success or major defeat, for if you have fought the change, it is usually evident here that the problem is going to become worse. If you have been fighting to save a failing relationship and transiting Pluto is in the last degree of your seventh house, for instance, Pluto's influence may cause you to make the decision to end the relationship once and for all, or be irretrievably stuck in a decaying situation. If the outcome is the former, congratulations, for you are now on your way to a new and better life. If the outcome is the latter, and you do not have the courage to do what should be done and end things, pray that Uranus will come along soon for the energies it represents will help you end it.

A similar burst of energy takes place at the early degrees of a sign or house, which has the effect of pouring forth an enormous amount of energy into a new area of your life. This is virgin energy, ready to be used in whatever way you will, and so brings with it tremendous anticipation and hope for a positive outcome. Therefore, when a planet enters a new sign or house, this is indeed an auspicious time astrologically speaking. However, the burst of energy at the final degree of a house or sign is a little more significant because it represents the final opportunity you will have to call upon that particular type of energy represented by the planet before it leaves.

ECLIPSES: WILD CARDS OF THE ZODIAC

If you have identified an episode in your life, a specific Jupiter or Pluto transit in which you noticed a significant weight gain, take a look at the eclipses that occurred at that time also. Symbolically, eclipses pack an extra punch and if Jupiter and Pluto were requiring any changes of you, an eclipse in aspect to these two planets would cause things to speed up. Eclipses represent intensity, so issues that are being surfaced will be placed prominently in front of your face; there is no denying them or running away from them. Their significance is similar to that of Uranus, but does not last as long. They can manifest in our lives in ways that can be just as disruptive as a Uranian transit can be. They are definitely representative of powerful drives that must be respected.

If you are open to change, you will probably look at eclipses as a good thing. You will realize that they are helping to make sure that the required changes are made in your life, and that whatever needs to be eliminated is eliminated. If, on the other hand, the change is perceived as something bad, then the energies symbolized by eclipses could make you miserable. Under normal circumstances, you can sometimes hold off a Pluto or Jupiter requested change, but if an eclipse is involved, you are almost certain to make the change, no matter how hard you may want to avoid it.

In summary, we learned that transits are extremely important in dealing with weight issues for two reasons. First of all, they highlight areas in our natal chart that need to be addressed immediately. Secondly, they provide the necessary impetus to tackle a problem once and for all. Transits of Jupiter and Pluto in particular signal opportunities to assist in ridding us of unwanted or outdated thought patterns and methods of living, or to step our consciousness up to a higher level of understanding. In this process, Jupiter and Pluto are aided by other planets. Neptune and Uranus are two planets which represent inner drives and motifs that complement the goals of Jupiter and Pluto, and can therefore assist in the elimination or enlightenment process, and Saturn is always a welcome friend when tackling any kind of tough project. Finally, we learned that with transits, timing is very meaningful, because these valuable planetary significances are only with us for a certain amount of time, and if we are truly serious and committed to making real progress, we want to take full advantage of any and all planetary help being offered to us.

If you have not already done so, this would be a perfect time to sit down with your chart and review the transits that are currently working in your life in order to assess whether or not you are taking advantage of the planetary help being offered. As a matter of fact, once you have identified the transits and the areas of your life being activated, try to determine intuitively how you can best use the symbolic significances of the transiting planets to improve your current life situation. The house in which Jupiter or

Pluto is transiting will indicate the area of your life being highlighted. Ask yourself if you are consciously able to articulate the change or elimination being required and how you are progressing. Even if you feel that you are not making progress, if you can at least determine what is being asked of you, then you are well on your way to being able to successfully handle the situation, for we all know that identifying a problem is the first step towards its resolution. If you are currently going through some rough transits, i.e., squares or oppositions, make a list of the obstacles as well as the adjustments you believe are required in order to work through the transit and use it to your best advantage. If you are having easier transits, i.e., trines and sextiles, identify those areas that are being aided by this smooth flow of the representative planetary energies.

Here is an example of a Jupiter transit. Suppose that transiting Jupiter is moving through the fifth house of creativity and that Jupiter rules the seventh house of our subject's chart. During the transit, it will conjunct natal Jupiter for about two weeks. Let's say that this person has always been interested in doing something creative with his spouse, but has never been able to find either the time or the money to turn this dream into something practical. The Jupiter transit would be an indication that now is the time to take action. In this example, the optimism and sense of expansion indicative of a Jupiter transit would be doubled when it conjoins natal Jupiter, which would result in especially potent inner drives, so our subject could make his dream a reality in a big way. However, if our imaginary subject were to hesitate out of fear of trying something new, then he could find that, at the end of the transit, he would be left with a few extra pounds representing the missed opportunity.

Here is another example, this time involving a Pluto transit. Suppose Pluto is currently transiting the ninth house representing, among other things, higher education and moral and spiritual values. Imagine also, that it has been squaring our subject's natal Pluto in the sixth house of work and service. This person probably would have been thinking about doing a different kind of work for quite a while, but has not done anything about it. With this transit, though, the urge to finally move out of her current work would be quite strong, and she would more than likely want to go back to school and educate herself, so that she could do something more in line with her current moral or spiritual values. Pluto transits work slowly, but are sped up when Pluto makes aspects to natal planets. Pluto transiting the ninth house is normally indicative of a gradual transformation of one's moral and spiritual beliefs, but by aspecting natal Pluto through the square in our example, the transformation would take on a sense of urgency. This individual would do well to listen to the advice of Pluto, that is to give up her old, unsatisfying line of work, learn some new skills more in line with her values and, therefore, increase her personal satisfaction and usefulness in the world.

If you have always wanted to make a Jupiter or Pluto type change, transits of these two planets signal that the time is now, and that there is help available. Timing is, after all, everything.

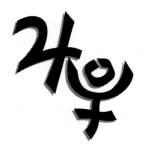

CHAPTER SEVEN

PROGRESSIONS TO JUPITER AND PLUTO: IT'S ALL ABOUT TIMING

In the last chapter, we looked at timing from the point of view of urges and drives originating outside ourselves, represented by transiting planets. In this chapter, we will again study astrological timing, only this time it will be from the perspective of symbolic internal influences and energies represented by progressions. Let's begin by looking at what a progression is and is not.

WHAT IS A PROGRESSION?

The idea that the planets have a symbolic influence on us as they move and travel through the various signs and houses of the horoscope was explained in the last chapter. When speaking of transits, we are referring to the constant movement of the planets through the heavens. However, progressions take this idea a step further. With progressions, we are referring to the movement of the natal planets in increments throughout one's lifetime; these planetary movements symbolize urges and drives which have an effect on us in much the same way as transits. The effect of progressions, though, is subtler than that of transits. Progressions are indicative of internal versus external awareness. What do I mean by that?

Let's take a person who has a preponderance of planets in the air and water signs. This person is normally pretty easy-going, not prone to anger. However, when she is age forty-five, her progressed Mars, planet of aggression, conjuncts her natal Uranus. Suddenly, this person becomes spirited, fiery, and volatile. She cannot understand why she is always angry. Something inside is urging her to say and do things that are totally foreign to her, and she cannot stop these urges. Now, had this Mars conjunction taken place by transit rather than by progression, she would have been warned by astrologers to be careful of arguments and violent people, things coming at her from outside herself. But with the progression, this anger and violent behavior springs from within and spreads out to whomever she comes into contact.

We can summarize by saying that while the end effects of progressions and transits are the same, they differ in the nature of the starting point of the symbolic energies. With progressions, the issues represented by the planets start from within, while with transits, they start from without. Other than that, one can interpret their effects the same way.

If both progressions and transits produce the same results, why do I separate them into two different chapters? Progressions, if handled correctly, can more easily create permanent change. In the last chapter, we talked about the fact that transits only last for a certain amount of time. Progressions also only last for a limited period of time, but because they work from the inside out, their significance on the psyche can be more powerful and lasting than a transit that is coming from the outside in. So, bottom line, if you want to make a change permanent, you have a better chance under a progression than under a transit.

There are two types of progressions, primary and secondary. They are both indicative of internal and external drives, so their symbolic effect is the same. Primary progressions, also referred to as solar arc progressions, look at each of the planets in your horoscope as if they moved one degree per year. Therefore, the aspects between the planets progressed by solar arc always remain the same; they simply change house and sign, but they do make aspects to your natal planets and to secondary progressed planets. These new aspects affect you in the same way as transits, except that their significance originates from within and works its way out.

Secondary progressions occur as your natal planets move from their position at your birth based on their speed of movement, that is, they use one day's normal planetary movement as the equivalent of one year in your life. The Moon is the fastest moving of the celestial bodies, and so the progressed Moon moves the fastest in your chart. The progressed Moon takes about two and a half years to go through each sign, so it will return to its natal position about every twenty-eight years. The progressed Sun, on the other hand, moves about one degree per year, and therefore takes about thirty years to progress through each sign. The farther out a planet is, the longer it takes to progress through a sign. Uranus, Neptune and Pluto hardly progress at all from their natal positions, and so don't have as much affect by progression as the closer, faster moving planets do. But if one of the faster moving planets aspects these outer planets by progression, this is an indication of a significant time frame for you.

THE IMPORTANCE OF THE
SECONDARY PROGRESSED MOON

The secondary progressed Moon moves so quickly, that it seems to function as a timer; its aspects to the larger planets, especially by conjunction, are major timing indicators in your life. When the progressed Moon conjuncts your natal Moon, this is an especially important time in your life, as it is an indication that you are now starting a whole new 28-year Moon cycle, and that you have internalized all that has occurred psychologically and emotionally during the last cycle. You are moving your life one turn up the spiral, and you are about to experience the entire zodiac from a new, higher perspective.

The secondary progressed Moon conjunct the solar arc Moon is also an extremely important time in terms of psychological or inner changes. As a matter of fact, anytime that the progressed Moon makes an aspect to a solar arc progressed planet, especially a conjunction, the qualities of the solar arc planet become internalized. For instance, if the progressed Moon conjuncts your solar arc Neptune, you have the opportunity to reach a heightened level of idealism or spiritualism. If the progressed Moon conjuncts your solar arc Saturn, certain karmic choices can finally be made, or you will be offered the opportunity to accept new duties or responsibilities.

This is an important issue for us in our study of weight control, for if the progressed Moon conjuncts your solar arc Jupiter or Pluto, there will be opportunities to finally internalize the resolve to either open yourself up to the mind-expanding experience of Jupiter, or to accept the necessity of eliminating unwanted baggage under a Pluto transit. Once you can accept and internalize an action, then you can perform it. If Jupiter has been pushing you to do something and you have been thinking about it, but haven't been able to bring yourself to act, a conjunction of the progressed Moon to your solar arc Jupiter will allow you to finally make the internal decision to act. The same would apply with Pluto.

The secondary progressed Moon aspecting any of your solar arc planets will mark the beginning of an internalization of the motifs of that particular planet. Even if it is not aspecting Jupiter or Pluto, the internalization of the motifs of any of the other planets can aid you in your efforts, as all the planets in some way deal with your personal and spiritual growth and development.

OTHER FACTORS AFFECTING BOTH TRANSITS AND PROGRESSIONS

Other issues that we dealt with in Chapter Six regarding transits are equally applicable to progressions. For instance, eclipses coming into contact with aspects involving progressed Jupiter or Pluto have the same significance as transits; the issues will be more intense and the action will speed up. However, the effect will be subtler with the progression. An eclipse conjunct your progressed Venus, for instance, could indicate an increase of activity in your love life, but the increase will begin by a change in your subconscious, as your inner attitude toward your love life changes. This inner change then becomes projected onto the outer world, and causes noticeable, physical changes in your love life.

As with transits, major progress can be made when progressed Jupiter or Pluto is in the last degrees of a sign or house. Additionally, when progressed Jupiter or Pluto aspects natal Jupiter or Pluto, this marks a time of tremendous opportunity; whatever area of enlightenment or area of elimination is being reflected by the planets receives an extra boost of energy, so major progress can be made. Finally, transits and progressions of the other outer planets, Saturn, Neptune and Uranus, occurring at the same time as Jupiter and Pluto progressions, can assist indirectly in the elimination or enlightenment process, so use them to your advantage.

CASE STUDIES

Now it is time to take a look at two case studies involving weight problems where progressions are involved. We will look at examples of both Jupiter and Pluto progressions.

CASE STUDY NUMBER ONE

This individual has Sun in Libra in the first house, Moon in Aries in the seventh house, and Virgo rising. She initially contacted me for a compatibility reading, but while we were talking, she happened to mention that she had recently begun to put on a few pounds and could not figure out why. Normally, she did not have problems with her weight, she told me, and her life had not changed, so she couldn't understand what was going on. Since I was working on this book at the time, her comments about her weight intrigued me, so I told her that I would take an in-depth look at her chart to see if I could identify any patterns.

Sure enough, I did notice something going on with Jupiter, both by secondary and primary progression. In looking at her horoscope at the time, the first thing that I discovered was that her secondary progressed Jupiter was in the first degree of her fifth house. In looking at her chart, keep in mind that the innermost ring in the wheel is the natal chart, the next wheel is the secondary progression chart, the third wheel is the solar arc chart, and the outer wheel shows the transits. Remember that any planet in the first degree of a sign or house sends out a huge burst of energy, so as to get us revved up to embrace the changes that will be coming our way as Jupiter makes its journey through that particular house or sign. It also gives one a very good idea of the kinds of changes to expect, which will be addressed shortly.

Her solar arc Jupiter was conjuncting her progressed Moon, so this was a significant time. The progressed Moon, remember, is an important indicator of timing; when it aspects another planet, especially by conjunction, it signals the start of the internalization of the process being brought about by the motifs of the planet involved. So when the progressed Moon conjuncts solar arc Jupiter, as in the case of this particular individual, it is an indication that she is beginning to internalize the expansion of consciousness related to the Jupiter transit, and if it is showing up as excess weight, it is more than likely because she is not yet allowing the expansion to take place in the proper way.

I am sure you would appreciate some background information on our case study, to better understand what is currently going on in her life. First of all, with her Sun in Libra and Virgo Ascendant, she is normally very easy to get along with, and quite refined in nature. This is reinforced by the fact that Neptune conjoins her Sun. However, if you rile her, she can show quite a temper for such a normally quiet woman. That is because she has her Moon in Aries, and Mars, the planet of aggression, is conjunct Pluto. This side of her nature doesn't show up very often, and over the years, she assured me, she has learned to handle these outbursts by simply going off alone until her old self returns. Her natal Jupiter, placed in her fourth house and trine her Ascendant, shows us a person who is very much in touch with her spiritual side, and the fact that Jupiter sextiles Venus is an indication of her normally optimistic and kind nature.

She told me that she comes from a large and loving family, and has always tried to pass on those feelings to others. She was married once, many years ago, but it did not last. She has no children, and says that the world is her child. She has worked in many professions throughout her lifetime, from bookkeeper to sales clerk, baker and probation officer. She likes being involved with people, working in groups, and her chart indicates that she does have some natural leadership ability where groups are concerned, as her Sun is sextile Mars and Pluto. She has not, though, used this natural leadership ability to any great extent, preferring to stay in the background, playing a supportive rather than a leadership role. The fact that her progressed Jupiter is moving into her fifth house is an indication that this is about to change.

Jupiter in the fifth is asking her to show off her creative side and to share her talents with the world. Jupiter is going to ask her to open up and let others know what she is thinking, and to take the lead in seeing that her ideas are brought to fruition. The idea of leading the charge had always been a little scary for her, reflected by her Virgo Ascendant; she felt as if she was not quite ready to take the lead. No situation was ever perfect enough for her. Also, her tendency to constantly weigh all the pros and cons of a situation, due to her Libra Sun, only added to her hesitation. She had been offered several opportunities in the past to assume a leadership role, but her super critical Virgo nature and her Libran indecision had always been enough to come up with a mountain of reasons whey she was not quite the right person for the job.

About two weeks before we talked, she had been offered yet another opportunity to head up a group of women working on a project for children. The group of twelve women wanted to do something for the local children's hospital. They just weren't sure what they should do. At the time, she remembered, she had many ideas about possible projects, such as making quilts, preparing toy or candy baskets, devising a puppet show, or even performing a funny play. When she mentioned her ideas to the group, they were quite impressed and asked her to take the lead in getting them going. Feeling that she was not up to the task, she politely declined. No one else volunteered to take the lead, and so they had tabled any action until they met again the following month.

The events of the meeting had haunted her for the next two weeks, and as we talked, she began to realize that it was around the same time that her eating had gotten terribly out of control. She said that every time she thought about leading the group, she would eat something. She also kept repeating that she could not possibly head up such a large project.

I told her that her progressed Moon was conjuncting her solar arc Jupiter because the universe wanted her to know that now was the time for her to begin her true work and service to her community. Her solar arc Jupiter was, after all, transiting her sixth house, and the planet of expansion wanted her to expand in that area. What better way than to head a group that would do wonderful, loving things for sick children? Deep down, I assured her, she knew that this was the right direction for her, and that she needed to overcome, once and for all, the mistaken belief that she was not qualified to lead. I reviewed her leadership traits with her as shown in her chart, the Sun in the first house sextiling Mars and Pluto conjunct in the eleventh house. I suggested that the reason that she was eating so much was because she was struggling internally with this new concept, the idea that she could actually step in front of the group and combine their energies to help bring her creative dreams in to reality. When we last talked, she had not made up her mind about what she would do, but promised that she would give the ideas we discussed some consideration.

CASE STUDY NUMBER TWO

This is an unusual case because the subject's mother, not the subject, is the person who initially contacted me. The subject is a male, and at the time was twenty-three years old. His mother came to see me because she was concerned that her son was going to self-destruct unless he changed his ways. She wanted to know what his future looked like astrologically, and what, if anything, she could do to help him. Her son, she told me, was extremely aggressive and always angry; he smoked constantly, used foul language, and was always intimidating the people in his surroundings. He had always been an over-achiever, had graduated from high school in three years, and recently completed law school. He was now going out into the world as a professional and was headed for disaster.

A look at his chart indicated that Pluto is quite prominent. (Note that in reading the chart, the innermost ring is the natal chart, the second ring shows secondary progressions, the next ring is primary or solar arc progressions, and the outer ring shows transits.) The chart was cast on the day his mother originally contacted me. Getting back to Pluto, first and foremost, it is angular, located in his tenth house of career and standing in the world, conjuncting the Midheaven. That by itself indicates an intense focus of energy on his career, and it sometimes indicates a tendency towards intimidating others and bending them towards one's own will. Having Pluto placed angularly in a chart would be sufficient to make it quite influential, but his Pluto also makes several important contacts by aspect with other planets. Besides conjuncting the Midheaven, his natal Pluto squares his Sun and Mars, sextiles his Ascendant, Mercury and Neptune, and semi-sextiles Uranus.

Also, his natal Sun conjuncts Mars, indicating someone who can be aggressive, blunt and rash in behavior. This, of course, confirms everything his mother had already told me about his hot-tempered nature. Additionally, his Sun and Mars, both placed in the first house, square his Midheaven, indicating an individual who is extremely achievement-oriented, and possibly someone who uses inappropriate methods to achieve their goals. Couple all this with the fact that his Sun and Mars are in the sign of Capricorn, again adding the desire for achievement, and you have a person driven by his ambitions.

The chart is all about control, and the use of one's will. From Chapter Five, we learned that possible meanings of natal Pluto in the tenth house could relate to power and how one uses it in their career or in the world. It looks like this person is going to have a lifelong struggle with these issues.

This chart by itself would not be sufficient to include it here in our case studies if it were not for the fact that his mother mentioned, in passing, that she was concerned about his health. He was smoking too much, she told me, and not eating well. He was graying prematurely, he was making a lot of enemies, and he was gaining a lot of weight.

Looking at the progressed planets at the time, you can see that his solar arc Pluto was at the last degree of his tenth house, and we know that that can be a significant point in the evolution of consciousness. Pluto was asking him to release his need to control everything and everyone, and to redirect, or transform, this energy so that it could be used in a more positive, beneficial way. At the time, his solar arc Pluto was ready to leave his tenth house and begin its journey through his eleventh house, and he was being bombarded with those transformational drives and urges, and was struggling to maintain his control of the situation.

What was actually going on in his life at that moment was quite interesting. He was just beginning a law practice, having opened a law partnership with a friend from college. They were struggling to obtain clients and build up a decent practice. His methods of obtaining clients were quite different from his partner's, and it was beginning to put a strain on their relationship. Since he does not believe in compromise, he was in a power struggle with his partner, and his partner had threatened to leave if they could not work things out. This concerned him because he had already invested a lot of money in this partnership and he did not want to have to start again with someone else.

He was fighting in the only way he knew, and the way that had always worked for him in the past, through intimidation and aggressive behavior. However, he was smart enough to realize that his tactics were not working this time, and he was concerned. As a result, he was smoking and eating a lot more than usual and his temperamental outbursts had increased. Curiously, at the same time that his solar arc Pluto was hovering at the last degree of his tenth house of career, it was also sextiling his natal Saturn. He didn't realize it, but he was being given an opportunity to change his old methods of operating and adopt a new, more appropriate way of dealing with others.

Unless he could recognize the opportunity being presented to him, it appeared more than likely that he would lose this fight. Notice that his transiting Pluto was squaring his natal Moon at the time, an indication that his basic, unhealthy behavioral patterns and responses were being unearthed so that he could face them and purge them. Power struggles would be especially tense at this time and, added to all the other Pluto issues going on in his life, could be enough to make him explode, or self-destruct, as his mother feared. Worse, unless and until he made the required transformation, he could make many more wrong decisions and thus cause his situation to worsen. At some point, a person exposed symbolically to this much Pluto influence by transit and progression should finally decide to make the suggested transformation, but because of all of his natal willpower indicative of Pluto urges and drives, he could decide to fight it for a long time.

I counseled his mother to talk with him in a non-threatening way, and to simply suggest possible modes of action. Someone struggling with as many control issues as her son, would not allow anyone to tell him what to do, but if she remained calm, he would probably listen to her as a trusted advisor. He, of course, would always make the final decision, which is as it should be. We cannot save our loved ones; they have to do it for themselves. We have enough trouble dealing with our own issues. In her son's case, he may have to "crash and burn" at some point in his life before he finally learns to let go of his obsession with control. If this does happen, as difficult as it may be for her to watch, all she can really do is be there to help him get back on his feet. The well-known power of the phoenix to rise from the ashes and soar to newer, greater heights lies within his grasp.

In summary, progressions, just like transits, are a major timing factor. Though their effect is more subtle due to the internal nature of the progression, once it is expressed outwardly, the progress can be the same, or even greater than the progress made with a transit. When we follow our inner hunches or urges, we always make the right choices, even though it may seem scary at the time. When Jupiter and Pluto urge us internally through progressions to make changes, we need to listen.

The princess was feeling very elated this particular summer after-noon, and she wanted to do something to express her joy. She was so happy, in fact, that she was bordering on giddiness. She threw her arms in the air and began to dance. As she danced, she began turning around and around in ever-widening circles. All this whirling and twirling made her dizzy, and finally she became so dizzy that she fell onto the soft, grassy ground in total ecstasy. The princess was completely unaware that while she was engaged in her happiness dance, Sebastian had decided to take a little nap and had lain down on the ground underneath a nearby tree. Unfortunately for him, he had chosen to fall asleep on the very spot upon which the princess fell.

The princess didn't realize that she had fallen on her little friend and teacher, until she felt something poking her back. She turned over quickly and saw that it was Sebastian. She was, of course, worried that she had injured or perhaps even killed him. She gently picked Sebastian up in her arms, and cradled him like a baby. He slowly opened his eyes, and gave her a look that quite surprised her.

"Put me down," he said, as if irritated. "And carefully."

She obeyed, shocked to see that Sebastian seemed to be perfectly fine. As he dusted himself off, she asked him if he was in any pain.

"Pain?" he looked at her incredulously. "Absolutely not."

"But you're a little elf, only two feet tall, and I am a full grown princess. My entire weight was upon you. Were you not injured at all?"

Sebastian gave her that look again, a look that implied total misunderstanding on her part.

"You did not hurt me because unlike you, I do not feel pain."

Having tended toward clumsiness all of her life, the princess thought that to feel no pain would be quite a valuable asset. She asked Sebastian to teach her how to do it.

"It is not anything that I can teach you," Sebastian told her, "but I know that one day, you will also be able to say that you feel no pain."

"How long do I have to wait before I can do that?" the princess asked. "Living a life free of pain would be very nice."

"And quite freeing," Sebastian added.

She didn't quite understand the correlation between pain and freedom, but had absolute faith that someday she would. In the meantime, she decided to continue with her dancing and promised Sebastian that she would be a little more careful of where she landed.

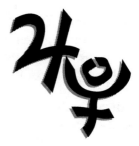

CHAPTER EIGHT

THE ASCENDANT: HELP OR HINDRANCE?

In Chapter Four, we looked at Ascendants in relation to our perception of reality and our ability to embrace change. In Chapter Five, we discussed some of the reasons why we are born with weight problems by looking at the symbolic significance of our natal Jupiter and Pluto. While you hopefully received many insights and clues as to why you have had a lifelong struggle with weight, this chapter will hone in on some specific problem areas. In this chapter, we are going to delve into Ascendants again, only this time, our focus will be on the role of the Ascendant in relation to physical traits and characteristics, including the tendency towards excess weight.

The tendency to be overweight throughout one's lifetime is related to the Ascendant because the Ascendant has much to do with our physical appearance. In addition to our perception of reality, the Ascendant shows how we present ourselves to the world, how we perceive ourselves and are perceived by others. There are certain Ascendants that are concerned specifically with physical weight, and these are the ones we will look at here. Taurus, Cancer and Leo Ascendants can perceive themselves in ways that call for them to present themselves to the world in a larger than normal way. Specifically, if you have a Taurus, Cancer or Leo Ascendant, you may be battling weight for your entire life, or until you realize the underlying reason for the weight issue and correct it. I want to take an in-depth look at these three Ascendants, analyze the causes, and offer some suggested ways of overcoming this problem.

Not everyone born with a Taurus, Cancer or Leo Ascendant will have a weight problem. There are many very slim Taurus, Cancer and Leo rising people walking around, which is an indication that they either learned to overcome the weight related issues of these Ascendants, or that they were never an issue in the first place. This discussion is for those who have those Ascendants and are plagued with weight-related problems.

Before we begin our study, though, I want to point out another related issue. If you think this chapter doesn't relate to you because your Ascendant is something other than Taurus, Cancer, or Leo, remember that your progressed Ascendant affects you as well. If your progressed Ascendant crosses into one of these three "weight" Ascendants, you may begin to have a weight problem where you had never had one before. If this is the case for you, then you should also pay particular attention to the following discussion. For instance, if you are a Gemini rising person and you have begun to have weight problems, it may be because your progressed Ascendant has moved into the sign of Cancer. Those with Aries Ascendants should do the same analysis, because when the progressed Ascendant moves into Taurus, weight issues may arise where none existed before. Those born with a Cancer Ascendant may have an especially difficult situation, as their progressed Ascendant moves into the sign of Leo after leaving Cancer, so they could possibly be waging a war on excess weight on two fronts. Since many of us will live long enough to have our progressed Ascendant go through several signs in our lifetimes, most of us will at some point have to deal with one of these three problem Ascendants. Again, Taurus, Cancer and Leo progressed Ascendants may not be indicative of problems for everyone, but for those of you who do have problems, read on.

One other Ascendant we will look at is that of Pisces. I saved the discussion of this Ascendant until the end because the reason for its inclusion is a little different from the other three Ascendants previously discussed. Pisces rising is included as a possible problem Ascendant not because it has a tendency to present itself in a large way, but because it has a tendency to exhibit traits of all of the other Ascendants, and therefore can, under certain conditions, resemble a Taurus, Cancer or Leo rising person.

TAURUS ASCENDANT

Depending on the degree of development of the individual, a Taurus rising individual can represent someone with unlimited wants and desires. These enormous wants and desires can manifest themselves as a huge physical body, especially if these desires are of a physical, material and earthy nature. The more material they are, the more they will show up as excess weight. Please do not misunderstand what I am saying. I am not passing judgment on Taurus rising people because they have a great desire or want for material things. Material things are fine, and we do all live in a material world and so we all have certain material needs in order to live. However, when we desire too much, or when we desire the wrong things, or when we desire for the wrong reasons, then we need to reassess our desires. Those Taurus rising people with weight issues might want to take a look at the nature of their desires, and perhaps make some adjustments. Perhaps you need to lift them to a higher level, i.e., instead of wanting a lot of material things, maybe you need to change your desires to social, moral or spiritual things. Perhaps you should examine your motives. If you find that they are a little too selfish, then you need to lift them so that they become less personal and more inclusive of others. If you lift your desires to a higher level, they become less "material" and therefore less likely to weigh you down.

Remember that we are looking at the significance of excess weight, the meaning behind the physical phenomena of fat. If you are a Taurus rising person, or your progressed Ascendant is in the sign of Taurus and you are dealing with extra weight, ask yourself what it is that you are desiring or wanting and how can you lift those desires to a higher level so that they are not so tied up with earthly wishes and more aligned with lighter, higher wishes.

Another reason that Taurus rising individuals sometimes struggle with weight is because of their close tie to the earth and the extreme pleasure they derive from things of the earth. They enjoy the beauty of nature, they love lustily, and they eat heartily. A beautifully prepared meal is highly appreciated by a Taurus rising person because it appeals to his highly developed senses. Whoever said "take time to smell the roses" was not addressing anyone with a Taurus Ascendant, because these people could write the book on appreciation of beauty, fine food and sensual pleasures. It is very easy to understand, then, how a Taurus rising individual could overindulge, simply because of his esthetic appreciation of the meal.

Appreciation of the sensual pleasures of life, including eating, is not bad in and of itself, and only creates problems when taken to extremes. The way to overcome this tendency is basically to follow the same advice given above. The nature of this sensuality needs to be lifted to a higher level. What I mean by that is that the sensual pleasures need to be replaced by higher-level pleasures. Sexual pleasures, for instance, which relate to our creative instincts, can be lifted to emotional or mental creativity. For example, you could paint a picture or write a book. Again, I am not saying that there is anything wrong with sex; I am just showing you how those same urges and drives can be lifted to a higher level or used for a different purpose.

Appreciation of physical food, then, can be lifted to a higher level by substituting food for the emotions, food for the mind, and food for the soul. Feed your emotional nature by exercising your ability to give and receive love. Volunteer at a hospital or homeless center, become a mentor, do something for someone else. Feed your mind by reading a book, studying a new profession, learning a new language. Feed your soul by doing something that will benefit your body, emotions and mind like taking up yoga, or learning to meditate. Feed your soul more and you will feed your physical body less. Of course, make sure that what you are feeding your emotions and your mind and your soul is appropriate. In the same way that we want to eat nutritional food, we want "nutritional" feelings and thoughts. Food for the soul should be uplifting and satisfying with an overwhelming feeling of peace.

CANCER ASCENDANT

Cancer Ascendants can have a problem with weight for a totally different reason than those with Taurus rising. Individuals with Cancer Ascendants can be extremely sensitive to the feelings of others. They are in tune with, or in touch with the masses, and can sometimes have a hard time separating themselves emotionally and otherwise from those around them. They usually have a strong desire to nurture others, and as a result, can have a very strong emotional tie to those under their care. And while this is a wonderful quality, if carried to extremes, they can end up having a very large "emotional field," so to speak, which can manifest in the physical world as excess weight.

To overcome this problem, the Cancer rising native has to learn to separate him or herself from others and develop his own individuality. He can still use his nurturing skills, but they should be delivered from the point of view of the fully evolved individual, detached and ready to aid others, acting as a complete person in his own right. He must not allow his extreme emotional sensitivity to color his reactions. After all, once he learns to know himself, he can then give so much more to others.

Another reason Cancer rising individuals tend to have more problems with weight than some of the other Ascendants is because they sometimes equate food with security. We've all heard the term "comfort food." A Cancer rising person probably invented that phrase. Security can be so important to this Ascendant, that overeating can be a subconscious method of trying to make sure that they will always be safe. Of course, food can never do this. Nothing can do this because we can never be totally secure. So how does one deal with this issue? By learning to embrace change. By trusting the universe. This is a tall order for those of you who have a hard time embracing change, and yet it is the only answer if you are substituting food for security. If you can learn to embrace change, you will no longer require security for you will realize that it is not only non-existent, but also undesirable.

In Chapter Four when we analyzed ways to overcome aversion to change, we looked at using the traits of the opposite sign to overcome that aversion. Since the opposite sign of Cancer is Capricorn, we extolled the virtues of that Capricorn trait of emotional detachment in dealing with the problem of fear of change. But while detachment will work when trying to overcome emotional sensitivity, it will not be as effective in overcoming a strong desire for security. Another Capricorn trait, perspective, will help shed light on many situations, including this one.

When one looks at a situation from a higher place, one can see many things that may not have been considered earlier, even though they have a bearing on the situation. From the emotionally insulated Cancer rising perspective, financial and/or emotional security appears to be the shell of protection that the little Cancer rising person needs to keep him safe from the outside world. But from atop the Capricorn mountain, one can see that the little protection afforded the crab by his secure shell pales in comparison to the other kinds of treasures available to him if he would only venture out. There is the treasure of freedom gained when one is true to oneself, the security of personal growth when one is open to change, the guarantee of truth when one faces one's fears. With all of those wonderful things waiting for you, why would you ever want to hide out in your shell of security?

LEO ASCENDANT

Leo rising people want to do everything in a big way. They tend to go to extremes. They sometimes celebrate just a little too much, may drink a little too much, often spend a little too much, and of course, eat a little too much. The Leo Ascendant has a big heart, and sometimes this big heart is expressed in an inappropriate way, resulting in an extra large physical body. The only way to handle this problem, then, is to redirect that big heart into more appropriate activities.

Too much love of self, too much love of eating, too much love of pleasure...I could go on, but you get the idea. All of this excess must be channeled into a bigger, higher cause. Too much love of self must be converted to include love of others. Too much love of eating and drinking needs to be channeled into love of giving, learning, creating and sharing. If you are a Leo rising person and you are struggling with your weight, ask yourself if you are a little too self-indulgent in any area, and if so, determine what you can do about it. We've all heard about that huge lion's heart, so I know that you are up to the challenge. Spread that Leo love around, lift it up to a higher level, and you will see that weight lift also.

Use that wonderful Leo quality of strength to improve the lives of those around you. Whenever we look beyond ourselves, we are able to throw off some of that self-indulgence or self-love which can weigh us down. That larger than life image of us will then shift from a large physical presence, to a large spiritual presence.

PISCES ASCENDANT

Pisces rising individuals can have more of a problem with weight than most other Ascendants for all of the above reasons. Pisces, as we discussed earlier, includes traits and tendencies of all of the eleven preceding signs. Therefore, the Pisces rising individual can suffer the problem of Cancer Ascendants by empathizing too much with others, being too sensual at times like some Taurus rising individuals, and going to extremes as Leo rising individuals sometimes do. If this is your Ascendant and you are having problems related to any of these issues, the cure is the same as we have discussed above for the Cancer, Taurus and Leo Ascendants. Assess the nature of your desires and determine if they need to be lifted to a higher level. Analyze your extreme behaviors and transfer the energy to a higher, more inclusive cause. Work on replacing emotional over-sensitivity with loving detachment.

So there you have it. Hopefully, you can see how these "problem" Ascendants don't have to be problems at all. For those of you who may feel that the advice given here is too ethereal or impractical, remember the discussion from Chapter One. Everything written here deals with significances and underlying meanings. The purpose of this book is to identify the underlying meaning or cause behind excess weight. Therefore, the solutions to these underlying causes will necessarily be ethereal and full of hidden or intangible meanings, so if you accept the premise that weight has an intangible meaning, it should be easy for you to accept the idea of an intangible cure.

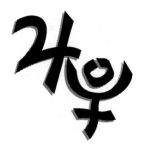

CHAPTER NINE

OVERCOMING PROBLEM ASPECTS AND PROBLEM PLANETS

In this chapter, I would like to address some specific problem areas that many of us encounter in our struggle with weight. There are certain aspects, houses and signs that are more prone to weight problems than others. We have already covered houses and signs and looked at possible meanings and solutions back in Chapter Five. And in the last chapter, we looked at challenging Ascendants. But now we are going to analyze problem aspects to the Ascendant. Since the Ascendant represents the physical body, Jupiter and/or Pluto in hard aspect to, that is, conjunct, square or opposite, the Ascendant can often indicate major weight issues.

The other area we will look at in this chapter is that of challenging planets. Referring back to the problem Ascendants in Chapter Eight, it only stands to reason that the planets ruling those Ascendants could also be representative of problematic weight issues. The Moon, because of its rulership of Cancer and its relationship to the emotional nature, the Sun, because of its rulership of Leo and importance to the sense of self, and finally, Venus, because of its rulership of Taurus and ties to the desire nature, can signify weight problems if in hard aspect to Jupiter and Pluto. Neptune is also being included in this discussion as a possible problem planet, as it is the natural ruler of Pisces. As pointed out in Chapter Eight, a Pisces Ascendant can include the traits of all of the other signs.

Jupiter in hard aspect to the Moon, Venus or the Sun can also indicate difficult aspects in relation to one's weight, because Jupiter's power of expansion implies excess emotional responses when in relation to the Moon, and the tendency toward over-indulgence when in relation to the Sun and Venus. However, as important as they are, these aspects will not be discussed here because we have already analyzed them in Chapter Five. If you know that you have one of these Jupiter hard aspects either natally, by transit or by progression, it would be wise to reread that section in Chapter Five, because the Jupiter/Moon, Jupiter/Venus, and Jupiter/Sun link to excess weight is incontrovertible.

Let's look at the symbolic significance of these problem aspects and planets one at a time.

JUPITER CONJUNCT, SQUARE OR OPPOSITE THE ASCENDANT

This can be a boon or a disaster, depending on the nature of the individual. If any one of these three combinations shows up in your chart and you are having weight problems, you should definitely explore its meaning. Jupiter in relation to the Ascendant is representative of an expansion of consciousness. Since the aspect determines how the issues symbolized by Jupiter relate to the Ascendant, having the combination in hard aspect indicates that there may be problems impeding the natural flow of these issues, and they need to be addressed. If you have this aspect in your natal chart, your entire life is one of continual soul growth. Obviously, if you do not have a natural affinity toward soul growth and change, you could be struggling with these issues your entire life.

Conjunctions are the most powerful of the aspects, for they represent a concentration of the drives and urges symbolized by the planets. A conjunction is very difficult to ignore; you will feel its presence. If you do not learn to come to terms with it, you could waste this wonderful opportunity to broaden your horizons and may simply broaden your physical body instead. A square between Jupiter and your Ascendant should alert you to the fact that there are obstacles standing in the way of your progress that need to be surmounted. Squares can be overcome; it is simply a matter of identifying the obstacle, making the adjustment, and moving forward. Oppositions of Jupiter to the Ascendant represent opportunities for compromise, for meeting in the middle. If this compromise takes place, the result is similar to the conjunction, for you then have the two planetary motifs working together, and the enormous power that it brings.

Examples of obstacles to be overcome with this planetary pattern might include an overblown sense of self, resulting in excessive pride. You may be overly optimistic and therefore lacking in judgment, or you could be prone to making promises that you can't keep. Overcoming an obstacle such as egoism or excessive pride requires that you learn to see all sides of an issue and that you consider the point of view of others. To do this, you must remove yourself from the center of the situation. One way to do this would be to seek out the opinion of someone you trust to give you an unbiased evaluation of the situation. Another way is to imagine yourself in the shoes of the other person and to see the situation from their perspective. If you are dealing with the obstacle of excessive optimism, you might try overcoming it by always making a list of pros and cons before reaching any major decision, rather than hastily forming an opinion or giving a promise. Seeking trusted advice works here also. There is nothing wrong with being optimistic or having confidence in yourself, but anything carried to extremes is not good. Jupiter squaring or opposing your Ascendant is a signal that you need to learn how to recognize the signs that you are going overboard in the optimism department and that you need to put on the brakes. However you teach yourself to do that is fine, as long as you are able to recognize when it is time do to so and have a plan that you can put into place. Your plan may be as simple as "sleep on it" in order to postpone action for a while. The most important thing is that you do have a plan.

If you are dealing with the aspect by transit or progression, rather than natally, you may put on tremendous amounts of weight during the period of this transit or progression unless you can identify and absorb the changes represented by Jupiter. The sooner you identify the issues and allow the mind-expansion to take place, the sooner the suffering ends. If not, the weight is liable to remain with you for a long time to come.

The kinds of issues you will be dealing with under these aspects are the same as those relating to Jupiter in the first house, discussed in Chapter Five. However, the issues are more intense when the Ascendant is involved. The Ascendant is one of the four angles, which are major points in an astrological chart, and any planet in aspect to an angle will have a major influence in the life to the individual. Along with the IC, Descendant and Midheaven, the Ascendant sets the tone for the direction of the individual in this lifetime. Any planets in aspect to any of the angles, have a profound symbolic significance on the direction the individual takes and the resultant achievements, failures, and lessons learned. Jupiter motifs are indicative of new perceptions of the world; allow this experience to happen and your life will be one of constant change, amazement and wonder. Fight it and your soul may atrophy, and this beautiful mind-awakening opportunity could deteriorate into an extremely heavy burden.

PLUTO CONJUNCT, SQUARE OR OPPOSITE THE ASCENDANT

Pluto in aspect to the Ascendant aligns its symbolic energies with those of the Ascendant to bring about the elimination process we have been discussing all along in this book. However, because of the powerful nature of the Ascendant, the eliminative process takes on a new urgency. This relationship of Pluto to the Ascendant in the natal chart tells the native that the elimination and/or transformation must happen in this lifetime if the individual is to live the life that the horoscope promises. If these aspects show up in your chart by transit or progression, you must look at what is currently happening in your life and understand the urgency of that particular transformational process.

The conjunction, of course, is the most powerful, and if this shows up in your natal chart, expect to live a powerful, intense life. If you have this aspect, you already know what I am talking about. There is so much intensity and focus and power in your nature that you probably feel that you can will things to happen. If this aspect shows up in your chart by transit or progression, expect the same kind of personal power for the period of the transit or progression. Because of the great power and resourcefulness that you possess, you can easily make the necessary transformations required by Pluto, and should be quite successful. Therefore, if you are a person with Pluto conjunct the Ascendant and are suffering with weight problems, you are probably misdirecting your personal power. You need to aim your power squarely at the root cause. Reread some of the possible issues that Pluto in the first house represents as outlined in Chapter Five. Then multiply them by ten, as Pluto on the Ascendant brings an added sense of urgency.

Pluto opposite the Ascendant requires that you look at the traits of your Descendant and try to incorporate some of those into your life, to achieve balance. The square is asking you to identify the obstacle, again, probably relating to a misdirecting of your drives, urges and motives, and make the necessary changes to overcome it. Examples of obstacles to be overcome or oppositions to be mediated with this planetary configuration might include a tendency to force your views on others, or to manipulate relationships for your own benefit. A way to overcome a tendency to force your views on others would be to accept the fact that there are certain things that you cannot change, and realize that sometimes it is necessary to simply step back and allow the universe to handle things. Since Pluto is involved, a release of some sort is necessary; what you need to learn to release is your desire to control others and to control all the circumstances in your life.

The advice for dealing with this set of aspects is basically the same as that when dealing with Pluto in general, only it is being shouted out this time to make sure you hear it. Figure out what it is that should be eliminated from your life and then eliminate it, or you may be saddled with an unfilled existence.

MOON CONJUNCT, SQUARE OR OPPOSITE THE ASCENDANT

The Moon is powerfully connected to your emotional nature and your psychological foundation. As a result, hard aspects to the Ascendant from the Moon are usually indicative of some deep-seated emotional or psychological issue that needs to be adjusted. Since it is related to the Moon, you probably have an instinctive understanding of what the issue is, and are more than likely overly connected to it emotionally. Conjunctions give you the most power to overcome these emotional issues, while oppositions and squares require you to work a little harder.

If you have any of these aspects in your natal chart, your life could be one of emotional or psychological instability that could manifest in a life long battle with weight, because this emotional struggle manifests as a struggle to maintain a balanced form. Transits of the Moon move so quickly that they are not really an issue because they do not allow enough time for much growth, but progressions are quite important. The progressed Moon, as explained earlier, is an important indicator of timing; if your progressed Moon is in hard aspect to your Ascendant, especially the conjunction, you are being told that it is now time to deal with the issue involved. You may have tried earlier and been blocked; this time you have the inner strength to succeed, should you choose to do so.

Examples of obstacles that you may have to overcome with the Moon squaring or opposing your Ascendant might include being extremely gullible, having overly emotional or subjective reactions to situations, or possibly conditioned emotional responses which are no longer appropriate. The best way to overcome these obstacles is to train yourself to look for conditioned responses and to stop them before they are acted out. A popular method is to count to ten when angry or on the verge of behaving incorrectly, so that you will have time to formulate a more appropriate response. As far as gullibility, this is the result of a totally emotional response to situations; one way to overcome this obstacle would be to try to approach situations from a mental perspective. Before making decisions or accepting what you hear as truth, ask questions. The act of questioning will take you from the emotional level to the mental realm and will allow you to see and understand things more clearly.

In order to overcome hard aspects of the Moon to your Ascendant, you need to look to the Jupiter and Pluto placements in your natal chart, and their transits, for this is when opportunities will arise to face your problem areas head on.

SUN CONJUNCT, SQUARE OR OPPOSITE THE ASCENDANT

The Sun highlights any problems existing in the area in which the Sun is located. In the natal chart, if your Sun is in hard aspect to your Ascendant, personal self-expression is highlighted. This could be an indication that you will have a problem with self-expression all of your life unless you learn to identify the root cause and overcome it; this usually takes place with a Pluto or Jupiter transit or progression. Until you are able to overcome or eliminate the issues, you could experience weight problems that represent the repression of your personality expression.

If hard aspects from the Sun to your Ascendant appear in your natal chart, your ability to develop a strong sense of self could be extremely retarded; if you are struggling in this area, know that you have the ability to switch from a negative to a positive self-expression in this lifetime. Because the Sun moves so quickly through the horoscope, having these aspects by transit really does not present much of a problem. But if they occur by progression, you will have two or three years where you will have to deal with these issues. Again, the answers will come by analyzing your natal Jupiter and Pluto placements, and by using the symbolic energies supplied by Jupiter and Pluto transits.

Examples of obstacles with this planetary configuration could include difficulty in making yourself understood, trouble relating to people, or general problems with self-expression due to a conflict between your true self and the self you present to the world. This can sometimes result in the feeling that you must bury your individuality in order to be acknowledged and accepted by others. An answer to this situation is to find out who you truly are, and integrate that into the self that you present to the world. You might try meditating or simply spending more time alone in contemplation. Make lists of your likes and dislikes in all areas of life, i.e., favorite books, tv shows, movies, favorite kinds of foods, favorite vacation spots, etc. and see what you can glean about yourself from that information. Ask yourself open-ended questions like what you would do if you were given a million dollars. Answer truthfully and you will begin to get a glimpse of what your values are, which are, after all, a reflection of your true self.

Finding out who you truly are is a difficult task, but Pluto transits can assist you in eliminating some of the things that are hiding the inner you from your outer self, and Jupiter can open up areas that will shed new light on who you really are.

VENUS CONJUNCT, SQUARE, OR OPPOSITE THE ASCENDANT

Venus in hard aspect to your natal Ascendant indicates problems with your desire nature, and can trigger the tendency toward overindulgence in the pleasures of life. Hard aspects of Venus are similar to those of Jupiter; they usually imply extremes—in this case, extremes of sensual desires. If you have any of these natal placements of Venus and are suffering from weight issues, the answer most likely lies in the nature of your desires. An adjustment needs to be made, and by looking at your natal Jupiter and Pluto placements, you should be able to get an idea of what should be done. The transits of Jupiter and Pluto will give you opportunities to do this work.

Examples of obstacles to be overcome or adjustments to be made with Venus in hard aspect to the Ascendant could include a tendency towards procrastination, being too easygoing or, because things come so easily to you, a tendency to be spoiled or lazy. Also, there can be difficulty in relating to others, especially in expressing love and affection. Suggested ways of overcoming procrastination, laziness, and over-indulgence would be to learn to desire less or to desire different things. Difficulty in relating to others is sometimes the result of placing your desires and needs ahead of others; simply thinking of the other person first will assist in changing your outlook and thereby overcoming the obstacle to personal growth. Venus is a very magnetic planet and can attract its desires to itself quite easily, so a shift in the kinds of things it *wants* to attract will create a shift in the kinds of things it *does* attract. Again, opportunities to work on these areas will abound under Jupiter and Pluto transits and progressions.

NEPTUNE CONJUNCT, SQUARE OR OPPOSITE THE ASCENDANT

Neptune is the higher octave of Venus and, as such, represents all of the qualities of Venus and more. Like Venus, it is extremely magnetic and, therefore, can attract love, money, and weight in the same way that Venus can. Its version is both more idealistic and spiritual in nature, or, if misinterpreted or misused, it can result in extreme confusion and disillusionment.

Neptune conjunct the Ascendant will, at its highest, be indicative of someone with a very lofty and idealistic vision of life and the world; at its lowest, it can indicate someone inclined toward escapist tendencies. The square and opposition are watered down versions of these tendencies and, once again, to reach the higher level of Neptune, you must identify and overcome the obstacle that the square represents, and use compromise to meet the opposition in the middle. Examples of obstacles could include an unrealistic outlook on life, living in a fantasy world, self-deception, extreme moodiness, sensitivity, confusion or faulty judgment. With the square and opposition, you may feel that you have difficulty grasping what is real and that you have no connection to anything solid or tangible. To overcome these obstacles requires some kind of grounding—emotional, mental, physical, or all three. If, for instance, you find yourself constantly making faulty decisions, force yourself to require more facts before making your next decision. If you find that you are lost and confused, seek counsel from those you consider wise enough to offer you straightforward, common sense advice. Choose someone with a proven track record, someone who has given you good advice in the past. You can also look at the examples that others have set who have been in similar situations and made correct decisions.

If you have Neptune in hard aspect to your Ascendant, either natally or by transit or progression, and are struggling with weight issues, the only answer in dealing with these energies is to force yourself to take the higher road whenever choices for change and transformation are presented to you. Opportunities to do this will arise under transits of Jupiter and Pluto. If you make the wrong decisions when these opportunities are presented, you could find yourself mired in confusion, unable to find your sense of direction.

Hanging upside down from a tree must be very tiring, the princess thought, but she was hesitant to express her conclusion out loud for fear of offending the little elf. After all, he must believe that this is an appropriate pastime since he does it so often. Indeed, the little elf seemed to hang from a tree whenever he was engrossed in deep thought or meditation, which usually occurred at some point every day. The first time she ever saw Sebastian engaging in this activity, she thought that something must be wrong with him, for when she asked him what he was doing, he didn't respond. In fact, he didn't say anything to her until he turned right side up again, some two hours later. She had learned to find other activities to occupy her time whenever Sebastian was meditating.

Today had started out like any other day. The sun was shining brightly over the beautiful valley, the river was flowing musically along, and Sebastian was hanging upside down from a tree. Everything appeared to be perfectly normal, but the princess was unaware of sinister goings-on nearby, that would eventually impact her and the little elf.

High above the princess, the elf, and the tree from which he was hanging, a large hawk was circling, looking for prey. The hawk was quite hungry, as he had not eaten a good meal in several days. From his perspective, Sebastian appeared to be a bright blue speck, misinterpreted by the hawk as some sort of fruit from a strange tree. The hawk would have preferred a protein meal, but he was desperate, and strange blue fruit was better than nothing. So, after circling the tree several times from the air, the hawk swooped down in a straight line, right towards Sebastian, who was still hanging upside down, deep in his meditative state. At the time of the attack, the princess was engrossed in studying the shape of her toes, and was therefore caught off guard. By the time she realized what was happening, the hawk was already within several feet of Sebastian. She screamed a warning to Sebastian, but he was totally unresponsive. Fearing the worst for her friend, she leapt towards him, hoping to grab him before the hawk could.

Misjudging the distance between her and the elf, she fell flat on her face, and when she lifted up her head, expecting to see the hawk flying away with her friend, instead she saw something quite amazing. The elf, still in his thoughtful trance, hanging from the same branch of the tree, appeared to be emanating some sort of invisible force field or shield that the hawk could not penetrate. The hawk had flown to within two feet of the elf and then appeared to hit something. The hawk then flew back to its starting point and swooped down again, only to stop again abruptly about two feet from the little elf. Over and over, this scene repeated itself, the hawk swooping down, stopping right before he could make contact with the elf, and then starting over again. After about the tenth time, the princess approached the hawk and asked him why he kept bothering the elf.

"It's obvious you're never going to win," she told him, "so why not just go on your way? There must be other, better prey out there."

"Quite true," the hawk agreed, "I've expended enough energy here." He looked as if he were going to fly away, then turned and asked the princess, "how do you taste?"

"Not very good, I'm afraid."

The hawk looked at her for a moment, and then decided that he would probably have better luck somewhere else, and flew away.

Sebastian had not awakened from his trancelike state in spite of all the excitement. The princess way dying to tell him all about everything that had transpired, but she knew from previous experience that she could not awaken him. So she stood next to him, eyeball to closed eyeball, impatiently waiting for him to wake up.

"Sebastian, you will never guess what happened to you," she blurted out, as soon as she saw movement return to her little friend. "A giant hawk swooped down from the sky and tried to grab you for his dinner, but every time he came within two feet of you, something stopped him. And you just slept through the whole thing."

Sebastian was silent as he stared into her excited eyes, and the princess wondered if he were questioning in his mind why she had not helped him.

"I did try to help you," she blurted out in her defense, "but I fell down."

"Don't worry, princess. I was never in danger," he told her.

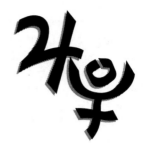

CHAPTER TEN

PUTTING IT ALL TOGETHER

A lot of information has been presented here, and you may need some help in putting it all together. This last chapter is an attempt to assist you in making sense of everything, and to give you a starting place in your personal journey to find the reason behind your excess weight. Once you identify the underlying reason for the excess weight, it is simply a matter of making the necessary adjustments. So, here is a logical, methodical approach to understanding and then solving your weight problem.

STEP ONE. Eliminate your fear of change. Place yourself in the mindset that all change is positive and should be embraced. If you are not able to stand in that place, then re-read Chapter Four. Unless and until you can see change as positive, it will be very difficult to understand the true meaning of your weight. Life is change. If everything remained the same, we would never grow, we would never be challenged, we would never be forced to face our demons and, as a result, we would never slay them. Another way of looking at change is to see it as freedom, for through the mechanism of change, we free ourselves from the obstacles that fear places in our way as we journey towards self-fulfillment.

Slowly and persistently, try to confront your fear of change. Realize that this fear is just an incorrect perception of the situation, and that if you can change your perception, you can eliminate your fear. Work on conquering that fear before you make any attempts to address your weight issues.

Suppose, though, that you have learned to perceive change as positive, but still have one or two other major fears standing in your way. The two most treacherous obstacles to progress are fear of the future and fear of failure. The key to overcoming both is to learn to live in the present. Fear of the future is based on trying to define the future based on the past, instead of allowing it to evolve. Fear of failure is based on the erroneous conception that failure is bad. Any past failures are of no importance now, except for the lessons learned. It is okay to remember the moral of the lessons, but it is futile and counter-productive to dwell on the past. And as far as the future (and any fears related to it) is concerned, how do you fear something that doesn't exist yet? The only reality is the present moment in which you are living, and the only time is now.

A mistake that can sometimes be made by astrologers is that they spend so much time looking at what is coming up in the future that they miss out on the present. Remember that if you don't live in the present, the future will not be what you want or expect it to be. The person that you see in the mirror everyday is the sum total of everything that has happened in your past. Whatever you did in the past cannot be changed or altered. The only thing that matters is what you are today. Live every day of your life as if it is the only day. Reward yourself every day, love someone every day, express your truth everyday, and the future will be exactly as it is supposed to be.

STEP TWO. If your weight gain is recent, go back to the time when you gained it and look at transiting, progressed and solar arc Jupiter and Pluto. Try to determine the exact time frame when the original weight gain took place. Then, look at the houses and signs in which Jupiter and Pluto were transiting at that time. Analyze the meaning of those houses and signs, and see if you can determine what it was that they were requiring of you and which areas of your life were being affected. What was it that Jupiter was trying to make you see? What was it that Pluto was asking you to get rid of? If you need help with this analysis, re-read Chapters Five, Six and Seven, as these chapters discuss the weight issues related to house and sign placement of transiting and progressed Jupiter and Pluto.

Next, check to see if Jupiter or Pluto were making any aspects to your natal or progressed planets during the transit. Again, check Chapter Five for insights into the meaning of these aspects. Ask yourself the same questions. What was the area of my life that Jupiter wanted to enlighten and how does that relate to the planet it was aspecting? What was it that Pluto wanted me to let go of or eliminate from my life in relation to the planet it was aspecting?

STEP THREE. If your weight has been out of control all of your life, closely analyze your natal Jupiter and Pluto by house and sign. Look at the aspects that these planets make to the other planets. Reread Chapter Five to gain insights on what it all means. Then ask yourself what it is that Jupiter is trying to teach you and what it is that Pluto is asking you to eliminate. If you have been having problems with weight all of your life, it is usually more difficult to ascertain the cause than if your weight problems started with a recent transit. This is true because if we have been dealing with an issue all of our lives, we may have learned all kinds of ways to bury it under mountains and mountains of other things, including weight, so that we sometimes have to really dig to find it.

STEP FOUR. Be honest with yourself. Most of the time, we know what it is that needs to be eliminated, or we know the area of life that needs to be enlightened, and we are just avoiding it out of fear of change, fear of the future, or fear of failure. Subconsciously, these fears stand in the way of our being able to face our problems, which is why we have to work on eliminating them. We have already discussed how to handle these fears in STEP ONE, and you should not be at STEP FOUR unless you have already dealt with all of your fear issues. Go back and re-read STEP ONE if you need to. Remember that once the fears have been removed, it is safe to bring those issues to the surface so that we can deal with them.

If you have already examined your fears, and you have honestly looked at your life in relation to Jupiter and Pluto, then you should know the truth and it is just a matter of doing something about it. So what are you waiting for? Maybe you've known deep down inside that the reason you are overweight is because you are too controlling in your relationships, or perhaps you are too engrossed in material things, or you tend to be too self-centered in your relationships with others and need to learn to be more giving, or more inclusive, etc. Or perhaps you stuff yourself to avoid feeling all the pain in your life or in the lives around you, or maybe you eat because you see food as a security blanket. I could go on, but you can define the issue for yourself.

Intuitively, you may know what needs to be fixed, and more importantly, you probably know how to fix it. If that is the case, just go ahead and fix it. You should now understand that there is no reason to be afraid, and there is no longer any obstacle in your path to progress and eventual success.

However, if after doing this analysis, you are still having problems determining what it is that you are being asked to change, here are a few things you can do. You could start by asking trusted friends and family members for their insights. Sometimes we can't see things because we are too close to them. Children, also, are especially good at pointing out basic, simple truths that we as adults sometimes miss because we are looking for more complex answers. Remember that the greatest truths are the simplest. The change may be as simple as changing your point of view.

Another thing that you can do to help determine the change that is being required of you is to ask yourself what you perceive to be your greatest weakness. Once you answer that question, see if you can intuitively correlate that with your natal Jupiter and Pluto placements. If, for instance, you perceive your greatest weakness to be your inability to make a decision, and your natal Jupiter is in the sign of Capricorn, then the answer might be that you need to learn to become more detached and less emotional in your decision-making process. If you feel your greatest weakness is your inability to stay focused on a single task, and your natal Pluto is in the sign of Gemini, then perhaps the universe is telling you to work on eliminating your tendency to be so scattered in your thinking and adopt a more probing attitude.

STEP FIVE. Be kind to yourself. Understand that change takes place slowly and gradually, and do not become depressed if you start and fail initially. You may have many false starts and periods of seemingly backward progress. But understand that you are making progress even if you think you aren't. The simple act of having the intention to clear up your problems is progress, and that seed, once planted in your subconscious, will eventually blossom into a full blown, manifested action if you only allow it.

Forgive yourself for setbacks. Allow yourself to dismiss the comments or criticisms of others that are contrary to your goal and your best interests. If you are in a stifling or toxic relationship, eliminate it with no regrets or guilt. If you know deep down that the change is good for you, then you must do it, and not allow sentiment to enter into it. Of course, you do not want to do anything to intentionally hurt anyone else, and you will want to make sure that you always take the high road. But often, that road is contrary to what others feel is in their best interest. Follow the truth in yourself, and you will always do what is right.

STEP SIX. Understand, accept and internalize the reason for the change. In order for change to be permanent, we need to understand and accept the reason for the change, and then internalize it. If changes occur in our lives and we do not understand them or the reason they were required, we will have a harder time dealing with our new circumstances. If, however, we understand why a particular change was necessary in our life, we will have a much easier time accepting and assimilating the change. What do you do if you do not understand why a particular change is necessary? Here is a helpful way to approach the situation.

If you know that you are being required to make a change and you cannot understand why, try looking at what will happen if you make the change. For instance, suppose you know that it is inevitable that your marriage is going to end. Your husband has told you that he is in love with another woman, and would like a divorce. You are fighting this because you still love your husband, and because you see divorce as a sign of failure. You have been gaining a lot of weight during this time period, and an analysis of your astrological chart indicates that Pluto is transiting your fifth house of creativity, and is opposing your Sun, the ruler of your seventh house. Jupiter is transiting your eleventh house of friends, groups, hopes and wishes. You remember that, years ago, before you were married, you loved to paint, but you gave all that up when you met your husband. If you don't fight the divorce, you decide that you would probably be very unhappy at first, but that eventually being divorced would allow you to become more involved with your creative side which you have neglected for quite some time. You allow yourself to believe that there may be a bright spot in all of this, which is that you may once again discover the joy you felt when you were creating paintings. Holding on to that thought allows you to make the transition from married life to life as a single artist.

STEP SEVEN. Accept responsibility for your choices and for your life. If you are still blaming your mother, or your fourth grade teacher or your cheating husband for your unhappy life, then you have not learned very much from this book. If you have read and understood the message of this book, you should understand that your life is your creation, and that the people in it are merely playing a part, the part you asked them to play, so that you could live out certain scenarios in order to learn and grow.

We all know that we attract people into our lives that reflect our current psychological state. We attract to us what we send out. If, for instance, you keep attracting mates that are irresponsible, perhaps it is because you are sending out the message that you are very controlling, and that you need someone to control. If you are attracting mates that are unfaithful, you might ask yourself what message you are sending out that allows others to believe that they can get away with cheating on you. In order to change the kind of people that show up in our lives, we need to change the kind of person we are. We need to balance our imbalances, and then we will not attract people who fill in the voids. If we can become a completely balanced person, we will attract other completely balanced people. Otherwise, we will continue to bring people into our lives who have the traits that we lack because we have a void that needs to be filled. We need to learn to fill in our own voids.

If you are overweight, it is probably because you need to do something differently in your life. It is not because other people treated you badly, or because someone left you, or because you make less money than your neighbor. It is not because you were passed over for a promotion, or because your parents loved your sister more than you. More than likely, you are overweight because you are clinging to an outdated version of yourself, and are refusing to change and grow. The reason you are overweight may be because you are not listening to that little voice inside of yourself that is telling you what you need to do to change your life for the better.

All of us have the power to change our lives for the better. I have given you hints here so that you can determine what needs to be changed, even though deep down you already know what it is. I have shown you how to overcome the fears that are holding you back. Now you no longer have any excuse. We all have a spark of divinity within, and this is the perfect time to find it, make friends with it, and use it. If your life is not the way you want it to be, and your body, which reflects your life, is not to your liking, then you are the only one who can change it.

CONCLUSION

"So how do I find you if I need help, or if I just want to talk?"

There, she had finally blurted it out. Sebastian had told her earlier that morning that he was heading for home today, and that she should now, too, be on her way. The idea of parting with her little friend saddened and, at the same time, frightened her a bit. The princess had tried to keep her feelings to herself, but could hold them in no longer.

"Close your eyes," Sebastian told her.

She obeyed, although she wasn't sure how closing her eyes would be of any help to her. By now she was used to Sebastian's unconventional requests.

"What do you see?" Sebastian asked her.

"Mostly darkness," she replied, sighing impatiently, still not sure where this exercise was heading.

"Look again," he demanded, adding, "only this time, take a few moments to think before you speak. There can be many things hiding in the darkness."

She closed her eyes again, expecting the result to be the same. But after a moment, she was able to make something out—something very small but definitely there.

"Okay, I do see a little bit of light in the corner," she reported to the elf.

"Walk into that corner and tell me what you find there."

The princess very carefully entered the small, lighted area and looked around. When she did, she made a most surprising discovery. While the lighted area had appeared to be very small before she entered it, once inside, she realized how very large it was. So large in fact, that it seemed to have no beginning and no end. It was just there.

"What do you feel," Sebastian asked her, "as you stand in that lighted place?"

"Why, I don't feel anything, really. It's as if I am floating in an unlimited, unrestricted space. I am very light and very free. I like it."

"And what do you hear as you float freely in this unlimited, unrestricted space?"

She was very quiet, and listened to the sounds of the lighted space. At first she didn't hear anything, but she remained quiet. Finally, she was able to pick up the sounds of the river, the whirring of the birds flying overhead, and the swishing of the leaves in the trees whenever a breeze blew through.

"And what of smell? Can you smell anything?"

She was surprised to report that she could, in fact, smell many of the fragrant flowers she had encountered on her journey with Sebastian. The roses, she told him, were especially fragrant; their aroma seemed to follow her.

"But I can also smell the apples we ate by the river, and the green grass growing next to the rock I sat upon when you were teaching me."

"And finally, what do you taste?'

That was a little more difficult to express in words. "I taste," she began slowly, "the sweetness of the apples we ate by the river, the tartness of the wind, the pungency of the smoke rising from the chimneys of the little houses in the distance."

"And what happens when the large hawk flies towards you and tries to take you to his nest and devour you?"

"He is repelled!" the princess shouted gloriously.

"And what do you see when you triumph over the hawk?"

She laughed. "Why, I see you, my dear friend. I see your smiling face and this beautiful valley, and the peaceful river, and all the birds and flowers that befriended me as we walked and talked here."

"And now that you have visited this lighted place, will you be dissuaded if someone tells you that it doesn't exist?"

The princess thought about it.

"No," she said emphatically. "Now that I know it is there, no one can make me believe otherwise."

"Even if they can't see it or feel it or touch, hear or taste it, they will not make you doubt its existence?"

"No, said the princess, "even if others can't sense it, I know it is there."

"And knowing of its existence, and having been there, do you need anyone to show you the way again?"

"No," she said, without hesitation, "I am sure that I can find it again by myself."

"Then," replied the little elf, "I am going home."

BIOGRAPHY

Beverly Flynn has been an astrologer for more than thirty years. She lives in Temecula, California, and is director of The Lighted House, a spiritual center where she conducts seminars and workshops on astrology and other metaphysical subjects. She also continues to do private horoscope readings. Beverly has been published in *American Astrology Magazine,* and is a member of the American Federation of Astrologers. If you are interested in learning more about her seminars, or if you would like a horoscope consultation, visit her website at www.thelightedhouse.org.

BIBLIOGRAPHY

Booth, Nicholas. *Exploring the Solar System*, Cambridge University Press, 1995.

Cotterell, Arthur. *A Dictionary of World Mythology*, Perigree Books, G.P. Putnam's Sons, 1980.

Hamlin, Paul. *Larousse Encyclopedia of Mythology*, Drury House, Russell Street, London, 1959.

Hathaway, Nancy. *The Friendly Guide to the Universe*, Viking division of Penguin Books, 1994.

Henarejos, Philippe. *Guide to the Night Sky*, Konemann Verlagsgesellschaft mbH, 2000.

"Jupiter in Astronomy." The Columbia Encyclopedia, Sixth Edition, New York, Columbia University Press, 2002.

Kaufmann, William J. *Universe - 4th edition*, W. H. Freeman and Company, 1994.

Motz, Lloyd. T*he Universe: Its Beginning and End*, Scribner, NY, 1975.

"Pluto in Astronomy." The Columbia Encyclopedia, Sixth Edition, New York: Columbia University Press, 2002.

Webster's Ninth New Collegiate Dictionary, Merriam-Webster Inc., 1991.

Also by ACS Publications

All About Astrology Series of booklets
The American Atlas, Expanded 5th Edition (Shanks)
The American Ephemeris 2001-2010
The American Ephemeris for the 21st Century [Noon or Midnight] 2000-2050, Rev. 2nd Ed.
The American Ephemeris for the 20th Century [Noon or Midnight] 1900-2000, Rev. 5th Ed.
The American Heliocentric Ephemeris 2001-2050
The American Midpoint Ephemeris 2001-2005
The American Sidereal Ephemeris 2001-2025
The Asteroid Ephemeris 1900-2050
Astrology for the Light Side of the Brain (Rogers-Gallagher)
Astrology for the Light Side of the Future (Rogers-Gallagher)
Astrology: The Next Step (Pottenger)
The Book of Jupiter (Waram)
The Book of Pluto (Forrest)
The Changing Sky, 2nd Edition (Forrest)
Easy Astrology Guide (Pottenger)
Easy Tarot Guide (Masino)
Finding Our Way Through the Dark (George)
Future Signs (Simms)
Hands That Heal, 2nd Edition (Bodine)
Healing with the Horoscope (Pottenger)
The Inner Sky (Forrest)
The International Atlas, Expanded 6th Edition (Shanks)
The Michelsen Book of Tables (Michelsen)
The Night Speaks (Forrest)
The Only Way to Learn Astrology, Vols. I-VI (March & McEvers)
    Volume I, 2nd Edition - Basic Principles
    Volume II, 2nd Edition - Math & Interpretation Techniques
    Volume III - Horoscope Analysis
    Volume IV - Learn About Tomorrow: Current Patterns
    Volume V - Learn About Relationships: Synastry Techniques
    Volume VI - Learn About Horary and Electional Astrology
Past Lives, Future Choices (Pottenger)
Pathways to Success: Discover Your Career Potential with Astrology (Geffner)
Planetary Heredity (M. Gauquelin)
Planets on the Move (Dobyns/Pottenger)
Psychology of the Planets (F. Gauquelin)
Spirit Guides: We Are Not Alone (Belhayes)
Tables of Planetary Phenomena, Rev. 2nd Edition (Michelsen/Pottenger)
Uranian Transneptune Ephemeris 1900-2050
Unveiling Your Future (Pottenger/Dobyns)
Your Magical Child, 2nd Edition (Simms)
Your Starway to Love, 2nd Edition (Pottenger)

The Electronic Astrologer
Reveals Your Future

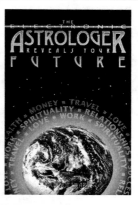

Three well-known and respected astrologers—
Maritha Pottenger, Maria Kay Simms, and
Zipporah Dobyns—have collaborated to write the
text for this predictive program. *Reveals Your
Future* interprets transits and secondary progressions to your birth chart and is written in an easy
to understand format. Full of insights, encourage-
ment and suggestions to make the most of any
aspect, you can be prepared for upcoming events
for yourself, your friends, or anyone you wish!
You choose the dates and *The Electronic Astrologer* does the rest.

There are 10 categories from which you can search; they include:
Identity, Communication, Creativity/Kids, Friends, Beliefs/Values, Money,
Home/Parents, Health, Relationships, and Career. Read the daily
interpretations as is, or click a button to see the aspects that deal with the
life area in focus.

Run progressions and transits singly or together; show aspects for one
day or print interpretations with a range of dates. Use predictive methods
with the most combinations available: transiting planets in houses, luna-
tions, progressed planets to natal planets, progressed planets to progressed
planets, or transiting planets to natal planets.

Features of *The Electronic Astrologer* include:
* Keyword Search • ACS's Unparalleled Accuracy
* Extensive Help System
* Built-in Atlas Database with Automatic Time-Change Information

The Electronic Astrologer Reveals Your Future   **IBMWEAF**   **$69.95**

Planetary Guide to Your Future

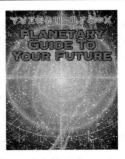

Prosperity, success, good health—all of the areas of your life are reflected in the transits to your birth chart. In Astro's best-selling report, *Planetary Guide to Your Future*, you will find vital information about how and when to make the right moves, which life areas will be in high focus during specific time periods, and constructive advice about when to pursue opportunities and how to achieve success.

Each month, you will learn about long-term transits and daily aspects to your natal chart, as well as the significance of each full and new moon. You can then choose the most constructive way to approach upcoming trends, make positive choices, and create the reality of your dreams!

A Planetary Guide to Your Future - 6 months (approx. 75 pages)	DTIX	$32.95
A Planetary Guide to Your Future - 12 months (approx. 150 pages)	DTIX	$49.95

Progressed Profile

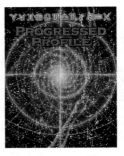

You have the power to create your own future—to take control of seemingly random events. Imagine having an outline of the year to plan your choices and decisions. The *Progressed Profile* gives you an advance look at the year ahead using secondary progressions. This reading offers you examples of the positive and negative ways in which you can approach each opportunity. Take charge of your future!

Includes a *Progressed Chart* that shows the progressed planet positions, the four major asteroids and Chiron.

Progressed Profile (approx. 15 pages)	PRP	$21.95

NOTES

NOTES